CARDIAC REHABILITATION

GUIDELINES AND AUDIT STANDARDS

Edited by

David R Thompson, Gerald S Bowman,

David P de Bono and Anthony Hopkins

1997

Royal College of Physicians of London

Royal College of Nursing

British Cardiac Society

British Heart Foundation

Acknowledgements

The work upon which this book was based was funded by a grant awarded to the editors by the Department of Health. The editors are grateful to the editor of *Heart* and the British Medical Journal Publishing Group for granting permission to reproduce chapter 8. The British Heart Foundation are thanked for a generous grant towards the editorial and printing costs.

The publishers are honoured that His Royal Highness The Prince Philip, Patron of the British Heart Foundation, has agreed to write the foreword to this book.

Royal College of Physicians of London
11 St Andrews Place, London NW1 4LE
Registered Charity No 210508

British Cataloguing in Publication Data
A catalogue record of this book is available from the British Library

ISBN 1 86016 0484

First printing 1997
Second printing 1998
Third printing 2001

Typeset by Dan-Set Graphics, Telford, Shropshire
Printed in Great Britain by The Lavenham Press Ltd, Sudbury, Suffolk

This book is dedicated to

Anthony Hopkins

The production of this book, though a team effort, was in no small part due to the vision of Dr Anthony Hopkins. As the book was going to press, it was with great sadness and sorrow that we learnt of his sudden death. We will miss his wise counsel, humour and friendship, and dedicate this book in his memory.

It may sound obvious, but the fact is that one of the very few parts of the body that is, literally, vital to life is the heart. The loss of most other parts may be inconvenient, but life can go on without them. Diseases, or abnormal conditions, of the heart are, therefore, very serious matters.

Thanks to the development of medical and surgical techniques, it has now become possible to treat these diseases and conditions, but, as with most other medical treatments, its success depends to a large extent on the process of rehabilitation. *Cardiac Rehabilitation; Guidelines and Audit Standards* addresses this aspect of cardiac care and brings together, for the first time, the experience of all the key professions. It reviews the evidence of the effectiveness of cardiac rehabilitation and this forms the basis on which the clinical guidelines have been developed.

I am sure that this book will prove to be very useful for all who are concerned with the provision of appropriate, effective and efficient services for the benefit of people recovering from heart problems.

Contributors

Gerald S Bowman MPhil
Research Fellow, School of Health, University of Hull, Hull HU6 7RX

Lorna Cay MD FRCP FRCPsych
Consultant in Rehabilitation Medicine, Astley Ainslie Hospital, Edinburgh EH9 2HL

David P de Bono MD FRCP FESC
Professor of Cardiology, School of Medicine, University of Leicester, Leicester LE3 9QP

Stewart Donald MRCP
Senior Registrar in Rehabilitation Medicine, Astley Ainslie Hospital, Edinburgh EH9 2HL

Alastair Gray PhD
Director, Health Economics Research Centre, Institute of Health Sciences at Wolfson College, Oxford OX2 6UD

Adrianne E Hardman PhD
Reader in Human Exercise Metabolism, Department of Physical Education, Sports Science and Recreation Management, Loughborough University, Loughborough LE11 3TU

Anthony Hopkins[†] MD FFPHM FRCP FACP
Director, Research Unit, Royal College of Physicians, London NW1 4LE

Michael Joy MD FRCP FACC FESC FRAeS
Consultant Cardiologist, St Peter's Hospital, Chertsey, Surrey KT16 OPZ

Alison Kitson BSc DPhil RN FRCN
Director, Royal College of Nursing Institute, 20 Cavendish Square, London W1M 0AB

Bob Lewin MPhil
Professor of Rehabilitation, University of Hull, School of Health, Institute of Rehabilitation, 215 Anlaby Road, Hull HU3 2PG

Andrew McLeod MD FRCP
Consultant Cardiologist, Poole Hospital, Poole BH15 2JB

Alan Radley PhD
Reader in Health and Social Relations, Department of Social Sciences, Loughborough University, Loughborough LE11 3TU

David R Thompson PhD FRCN
Professor of Nursing, School of Health, University of Hull, Hull HU6 7RX

Iain Todd MD MRCP
Consultant in Rehabilitation Medicine, Astley Ainslie Hospital, Edinburgh EH9 2HL

[†]Deceased

Contents

Editors' introduction

The Royal College of Physicians, The Royal College of Nursing and the British Cardiac Society have collaborated in producing this book, which reviews the evidence of the effectiveness of cardiac rehabilitation, and provides guidelines and audit standards which have been developed on this basis.

The volume comprises an edited and updated version of the papers first presented at a workshop held in October 1994, in which the contributors explore some of the important issues relating to cardiac rehabilitation. Dr Ian Todd and Dr Lorna Cay provide a useful and timely overview of work in this field, and point out that the task now is to agree on the important components of the rehabilitation process and to ensure that they are delivered at the appropriate time and in the most appropriate setting.

Dr Andrew McLeod reviews the medical goals of cardiac rehabilitation, programme management, efficacy and logistics, emphasising the importance of including a clinician in the rehabilitation team.

The psychological aspects of rehabilitation are discussed by Professor Bob Lewin, who stresses the importance of assessment and the evidence attesting to the efficacy of some simple early interventions to improve outcome. Dr Alan Radley examines the relatively neglected social aspects of rehabilitation, and gives a reminder of the importance of factors such as the social context in which patients and families operate and the role of social support.

The physiological and metabolic adaptations which result in improved functional capacity and endurance are described by Dr Adrianne Hardman, who also considers the efficacy, safety and applicability of different approaches to exercise training. Dr Michael Joy and Dr Stewart Donald present an overview of the vocational aspects of rehabilitation, including fitness standards and return to work, and emphasise the importance of vocational assessment and guidance. The different techniques of economic evaluation are outlined by Dr Alastair Gray, who points to the paucity of cost studies in the field of cardiac rehabilitation, especially in the UK.

The book concludes with a chapter on guidelines and audit standards, and an appendix comprising audit proformas. (This chapter has also been published separately[1] and is reproduced here by kind permission.)

Finally, we are greatly indebted to HRH The Prince Philip, Patron of the British Heart Foundation, for contributing the foreword to this book.

We hope that these collected papers will supply purchasers and providers of health care with evidence on which they can base clinical and service management decisions.

David R Thompson
Professor of Nursing, School of
Health, University of Hull

Gerald S Bowman
Research Fellow, School of Health,
University of Hull

David P de Bono
Professor of Cardiology, School of
Medicine, University of Leicester

Anthony Hopkins
Director, Research Unit, Royal College
of Physicians of London

Reference
1. Thompson DR, Bowman GS, Kitson AL, de Bono DP, Hopkins A. Cardiac rehabilitation in the United Kingdom: guidelines and audit standards. *Heart* 1996;75:8993

1 Overview

Iain Todd
Consultant in Rehabilitation Medicine, Astley Ainslie Hospital, Edinburgh

Lorna Cay
Consultant in Rehabilitation Medicine, Astley Ainslie Hospital, Edinburgh

To those of us who work in the field of cardiac rehabilitation, it has long been a paradox that we should have struggled for over 30 years to convince our colleagues of its value while almost every new treatment is grasped with evangelical enthusiasm by cardiologists. There is a further irony in the realisation that perhaps the greatest impetus to the expansion of cardiac rehabilitation in this country was provided by meta-analyses of the effectiveness of cardiac rehabilitation on cardiac mortality.[1,2] These studies were clearly valuable, although statistically open to question, and demonstrated the magic 20% reduction in mortality by which all cardiac interventions are judged, and in so doing gave rehabilitation a credibility previously lacking. The irony is that this should happen when it is beginning to be appreciated that hard end-points like mortality are not the only measures by which to assess the outcome of cardiological interventions. A move towards quality of life and cost-effectiveness assessments may lead both to a less mechanistic, more holistic approach to patient management and also to a greater appreciation of the value of cardiac rehabilitation.

With this in mind, it is opportune to evaluate the current state of cardiac rehabilitation. Such an evaluation should begin with a consideration of the history of the specialty, since that history has shaped its development. It should also consider:

- the changes which have taken place over the 30 years because they demonstrate where experience and research have indicated the need for change,

- where we are at present and, most importantly,

- where we should be in five years' time.

The aim of this working party, whose discussions form the content of this book, was to produce guidelines and audit measures for

those who currently run or are setting up rehabilitation programmes, with such guidelines tailored to future needs and not tied
to the past.

Historical conditions

The early management of myocardial infarction (MI) was characterised by prolonged bed-rest and careful monitoring of the patient.
It is little wonder that in such a setting the patient became physically
and psychologically debilitated. Recognising that patients often
failed to make a satisfactory recovery despite surviving the acute
event, a few cardiologists began in the 1950s and 1960s to develop
the concept of cardiac rehabilitation. Given the above situation, the
emphasis not unnaturally was very much on physical rehabilitation.[3-7]
Furthermore, because the problem appeared to be a failure of
relatively fit young men with uncomplicated infarcts to recover as
expected and concerns over the safety of exercise, particularly for
more complex cases, these early programmes were applied to low-
risk individuals in a highly monitored hospital setting. Research
suggested the need for two or three moderately intensive training
sessions a week of about an hour — and the pattern for programmes
was set.[8] Indeed, there are still classes today where little has changed.

It became apparent in the 1970s that rehabilitation was failing to
meet the needs both of patients and of society. While improvements
in work capacity could be related to exercise training, such improvements did not translate into everyday life, particularly in areas like
return to work.[9] Long-term compliance with exercise was found to be
poor, and high levels of anxiety and depression persisted.[10,11] For rehabilitation to be effective, clearly it had to be comprehensive. This
meant dealing not only with the physical needs of the patient but also
with the psychological and social needs. Patients and spouses needed
information about the disease, its effects, how it might be treated, and
its prognosis. Patients also needed advice on return to normal activities, and help with persisting anxiety to allow them to make a more
satisfactory recovery. Alongside the exercise component, this concept
of 'comprehensive rehabilitation' included educational sessions,
relaxation therapy and individual counselling. With the growth in
coronary artery surgery, it also became clear that many of the things
which held back the post-MI patient were equally applicable to the
post-coronary artery bypass graft patient,[12] and cardiac rehabilitation
programmes were then adapted to accommodate these patients too.

Comprehensive rehabilitation was clearly a move in the right
direction, but throughout the 1980s it remained tied by the rules

imposed on early programmes. Early-phase rehabilitation focused on information giving and early mobilisation, leading to such changes as the appointment of cardiac liaison nurses, but the intermediate phase failed to change because of the persisting belief that exercise was somehow dangerous and required specialist facilities. At a time when early mobilisation removed much of the iatrogenic debility of previous treatment regimens, and thrombolytics shortened the time course of acute MI, outpatient programmes continued to be dominated by exercise programmes along the previous rigid lines. By the close of the 1980s, however, there were signs of a change in attitudes. Research began to include programmes for patients with complications such as angina pectoris[13] and cardiac failure.[14] Such programmes were exciting, in that they challenged the traditional role of exercise as a tool for maximising recovery in asymptomatic individuals, seeing it rather as a therapy to improve symptoms in patients who would previously have been excluded from treatment. The success of exercise therapy in these patients is so much more tangible because of the change which can be brought about in the control of their symptoms.

The 1990s have added a new dimension to the rehabilitation process in the form of secondary prevention. We no longer believe that the die is cast with respect to prognosis. There are drugs which can reduce the likelihood of a further infarct, and fresh impetus has been given to the concept of lifestyle changes by trials of lipid-lowering treatments in individuals with established disease. The aforementioned meta-analyses have even given a boost to exercise as a beneficial lifestyle change. The most recent World Health Organisation definition of cardiac rehabilitation is:

> the sum of activities required to influence favourably the underlying cause of the disease, as well as to ensure the patients the best possible physical, social and mental conditions so that they may, by their own efforts, preserve or resume when lost, as normal a place as possible in the life of the community. Rehabilitation cannot be regarded as an isolated form of therapy, but must be integrated with the whole of treatment of which it forms only one facet.[15]

Future prospects

The challenge for the next decade is to integrate rehabilitation into an increasingly complex management strategy for ischaemic heart disease. The various components of comprehensive rehabilitation have been identified. We are aware of the problems which exist for the patient with coronary heart disease, and believe we have some of the solutions. We need to decide how best to apply these solutions and, by a process of continuing research and audit, develop a more effective and widely applicable form of rehabilitation than is currently the case.

Rehabilitation must begin at the point of diagnosis, and the cornerstone of that rehabilitation should be patient education. This is an area where integration of the rehabilitation process must be a priority. We are aware of the problems created by lack of information and, more importantly, by inconsistency of information. The patients' actions will be determined by their beliefs, some of which are pre-existing and others are created by what is said and done during treatment.

Clinicians must accept responsibility for providing effective information and for auditing the process, and they must ensure that all staff are consistent in providing information. This includes paying more than lip-service both to the process of information giving and to its documentation. An increase in time spent on interventions has undoubtedly reduced the time spent talking to patients — to the point that junior staff are fast becoming highly skilled technicians with poorly developed communication skills. In coronary care units, the liaison nurse may redress the balance — until a bright young registrar on a ward round suggests that the patient 'takes things easy' after discharge or hints that an angioplasty might be necessary in the future. Equally, the liaison nurse who writes in the case notes that advice has been given without stating the nature of that advice is not being effective. One of the greatest challenges for the next few years is to get this apparently simple process right amid an increasingly complex treatment strategy.

In considering the importance of patient education, the other patient groups should not be forgotten, including those with angina or cardiac failure who are often seen initially as outpatients. These patients often miss out on education, save for a brief discussion with a busy clinician. It is likely that the approach taken at that time plays an important part in determining whether the patient goes on to require angioplasty or surgery.

The rehabilitation process should include an assessment of the individual's needs and a treatment programme tailored to those needs, in the same way as the medical management of the post-MI patient involves assessment, usually at six weeks, and an individual approach according to guidelines. It is likely that with such a process we will stop prescribing exercise programmes blindly to individuals who do not need them, and free up space and time to prescribe them to those who do, including patients with impaired exercise tolerance due to angina or poor left ventricular function. It may then be possible to shape our exercise programmes to the needs of the patient by offering, for example, training for activities related to the patient's work or social activities.

For those patients for whom exercise needs to be encouraged simply as a lifestyle change, it is appropriate for such exercise to be community-based. We should therefore work to move 'routine' rehabilitation in that direction, encouraging appropriate patients to exercise outwith the hospital environment at an earlier stage without the need to 'graduate' from a cardiac programme. Supervision of this phase of rehabilitation should lie with primary care, and will necessitate improved communication between cardiac units and primary care. If successfully applied, perhaps the majority of patients who make up current hospital-based exercise groups could be moved to community-based rehabilitation, being replaced there by individuals of higher risk and greater potential benefit.

Patient assessment will also allow us to identify and focus on those with ongoing anxiety and depression in order to develop more effective and focused stress management, relaxation, or individual treatment. We are aware of the need for such treatments but, rather like exercise, the tendency has been to apply them too widely and sometimes ineffectively. Similarly, it should be possible to focus attention on those groups with special needs, such as individuals who wish to return to work, women, ethnic groups, etc.

Finally, programmes in future will consider the question of secondary prevention. The role of the rehabilitation team in this area may be twofold:

1. The team may adopt an assessment and advice role to provide the patient and general practitioner with information, on the basis that a long-term strategy for risk management should be the role of the primary care team.

2. Effective treatment strategies may be developed in the form of behavioural interventions for those patients for whom advice has not been sufficient. This is an area in need of research.

Summary

As rehabilitationists, we have made significant advances in the last 30 years. Many of the changes have been slow because of excessive caution on our part, and lack of support for the concept from others. A clear opportunity now exists to establish guidelines for rehabilitation, in the expectation that they will be observed, for the following reasons:

- more clinicians appreciate the value of rehabilitation;

- research is proving its value; and

- purchasers and patients demand it.

The task now is to agree on the important components of the rehabilitation process, to individualise that process and integrate it into both specialist and primary care so that the right patients receive the right elements at the most appropriate time and in the most appropriate setting. When this has been achieved, cardiac rehabilitation will have come of age.

References

1. Oldridge NB, Guyatt GH, Fischer MD, Rimm AA. Cardiac rehabilitation after myocardial infarction: combined experience of randomised clinical trials. *Journal of the American Medical Association* 1988;**260**:945–50.

2. O'Connor GT, Buring JE, Yusuf E, Goldhaber SZ, *et al.* An overview of randomised controlled trials of rehabilitation with exercise after myocardial infarction. *Circulation* 1989;**80**:234–44.

3. Levine SA, Lown B. 'Armchair' treatment of acute coronary thrombosis. *Journal of the American Medical Association* 1952;**148**:1365–9.

4. Newman L, Andrews M, Koblish M. Physical medicine and rehabilitation in acute myocardial infarction. *Archives of Internal Medicine* 1952;**89**:552–61.

5. Cain HD, Frasher WG, Stivelman R. Graded activity program for safe return to self-care after myocardial infarction. *Journal of the American Medical Association* 1961;**177**:111–5.

6. Goble AJ, Adey GM, Bullen JF. Rehabilitation of the cardiac patient. *Medical Journal of Australia* 1963;**2**:975–82.

7. Hellerstein HK. Exercise therapy in coronary heart disease. *Bulletin of the New York Academy of Medicine* 1968;**44**:1208–47.

8. Pollock ML. The quantification of endurance training programs. In: Wilmore JH (ed). *Exercise and sports sciences reviews*, vol 1. New York: Academic Press, 1973.

9. Nagle R, Gangota R, Picton-Robinson I. Factors influencing return to work after myocardial infarction. *Lancet* 1971;**ii**:454–6.

10. Cay EL, Vetter NJ, Philip AE, Dugard P. Psychological status during recovery from an acute heart attack. *Journal of Psychosomatic Research* 1972;**16**:425–35.

11. Cay EL, Vetter NJ, Philip AE, Dugard P. Return to work after a heart attack. *Journal of Psychosomatic Research* 1972;**16**:231–43.

12. Oberman AL, Wayne JB, Kouchoulios NT, Charles ED, *et al.* Employment status after coronary artery bypass surgery. *Circulation* 1982;**65**:115–9.

13. Todd IC, Ballantyne D. The anti-anginal efficacy of exercising training: a comparison with beta-blockade. *British Heart Journal* 1990;**64**:14–9.

14. Coats AJS, Adamopoulos S, Meyer TE, Conway J, Sleight P. Effects of physical training in chronic heart failure. *Lancet* 1990;**335**:63–6.

15. World Health Organisation. *Needs and action priorities in cardiac rehabilitation and secondary prevention in patients with CHD.* Geneva: WHO Regional Office for Europe, 1993.

2 The medical component

Andrew McLeod

Consultant Cardiologist, Poole Hospital

Overviews of cardiac rehabilitation have concluded that evidence of survival benefit is seen for patients who participate in exercise-based and multi-interventional programmes compared with control patients.[1,2] The mechanism of benefit is unclear, but sceptics of such programmes tend to attribute the improvements to better surveillance of cardiac patients. If this is so, it emphasises the importance of good medical practice in the management of patients. Increased patient contact with health care personnel is likely to improve the chances of correct management of medical problems which could jeopardise the patient's chance of survival. Coronary heart disease (CHD) patients are subject to sudden deterioration, even when seemingly clinically stable, and prompt institution of correct therapy is often important. Additionally, regular assessment and modification of therapy for other vascular conditions, such as hypertension, which impact on both coronary event risk and indirectly related conditions, such as stroke, are likely to be beneficial.

Medical goals of cardiac rehabilitation

The medical goals of cardiac rehabilitation have been summarised by the World Health Organisation as follows:[3]

- the prevention of cardiac death,

- decrease in cardiac morbidity (eg reduced incidence of myocardial infarction (MI) and coronary artery bypass graft (CABG) closure), and

- relief of symptoms (eg angina, breathlessness).

The medical input required to achieve these goals can be conveniently considered under four headings:

1. Risk stratification.

2. Further diagnostic testing and intervention.

3. Therapeutics and risk factor modification.

4. Programme management, efficacy and logistics.

Risk stratification

Mortality after first infarction is known to depend on several variables, the most important of which is the size of the index infarct.[4] A wide variety of non-invasive testing measures can predict additional risk. There is considerable confidence, though little firm evidence, that interventions, principally CABG surgery and percutaneous transluminal coronary angioplasty (PTCA), can modify this risk. Multiple methods of assessment can predict problems such as early recurrent ischaemia with risk of reinfarction, additional coronary artery stenoses in vessels other than the vessel of the index infarct, and the risk of arrhythmias. Unfortunately, the positive predictive value is poor for most of these tests.

The *negative* predictive value, however, is high.[5] This means that a patient without demonstration of complications from the index infarct, who has good effort tolerance, and is free from evidence of ischaemia, symptoms and ventricular impairment, will do well and remain at low risk, often for a number of years.[6] Cardiac rehabilitation programmes often include such patients, many of whom are also motivated to modify the risk factors which originally contributed to their disease. It is difficult to demonstrate in these patients that the programme enhances their likelihood of long-term survival.

In the UK, risk stratification is most commonly performed by exercise electrocardiography (ECG) alone, although additional prognostic information may be obtained by radionuclide perfusion imaging combined with functional testing.[7] The post-infarction ECG presents difficulties of interpretation during exercise.[8] Routine radionuclide study would probably be impossible for all post-infarction patients in the UK. The majority of cardiac rehabilitation programmes use exercise ECG testing, both as an aid to find the patient who requires further evaluation by coronary angiography or who is unsuitable at that point in time for inclusion in such a programme, and also to determine exercise prescription, which should be individualised for each patient.[9]

There is controversy over even this aspect of the medical screening process. Early exercise testing may pick up the patient with important recurrent myocardial ischaemia, and later — often higher intensity — testing may identify additional patients at risk.[10]

Exercise prescription is best made with the patient on the long-term treatment of choice (eg beta-blockade). Treatment with such drugs may mask ischaemia, although there is evidence that ischaemia which is apparent while on treatment is of more serious prognostic significance.[11] Pragmatism dictates that exercise testing while on therapy is valuable.

The concept of exercise testing following MI treated with thrombolytic drugs has recently been challenged.[12] There is presumably considerable hazard in the short term from the patent but still stenosed coronary artery. The evidence that over the next three years thrombolysed patients demonstrate a higher reocclusion rate than non-thrombolysed patients does not explain why the mortality curves in thrombolytic studies do not converge as time goes on.[13] The risk of reclosure may then depend on haemostatic variables which are unpredictable, at least by exercise testing. Such an assertion, however, is usually made after examination of short-term follow-up data. One of the strongest predictors of long-term risk remains the number of coronary vessels affected.[8] It is likely that some form of functional assessment will remain the cornerstone of techniques designed to identify patients at greatest risk, especially as both left ventricular function and exercise capacity are additionally predictive of outcome.

Whatever technique is applied to the assessment of the post-MI patient or the patient with CHD in general, the interaction of cardiac rehabilitation personnel with the patient and the physician responsible for the patient's care is likely to remain important in determining optimum therapy for that patient.

Further diagnostic testing and intervention

Coronary angiography has been proposed as the appropriate further investigation in the majority (probably about 80%) of post-MI patients. This policy, advocated by Kulick and Rahimtoola,[8] is not practicable in the UK, but it is important to examine the possible advantages which such an approach may confer.

Although coronary angiography combined with left ventriculography can enhance diagnostic precision, it is probably of definite benefit only to the patient with operable three-vessel CHD or left main CHD. The significance of a severe residual stenosis in the infarct-related artery is still debated. Trials designed to determine possible benefit of intervention, such as the Thrombolysis in Myocardial Infarction (Phase IIB) (TIMI IIB) and the Should We Intervene Following Thrombolysis (SWIFT) trials, did not demonstrate any utility of routinely revascularising such lesions.[14,15]

From the point of view of the rehabilitation patient, however, the value of such an approach lies in optimisation of the patient's risk before he or she enters the rehabilitation programme. Both the early exercise assessment and the additional surveillance of cardiac rehabilitation staff in the early phases of an inpatient or outpatient programme may help to identify the patient who needs invasive investigation.

Revascularisation by CABG or PTCA is continuously improving technically. Recent overviews of long-term results of CABG confirm that a clear difference exists in the fate of patients with left main coronary artery stenosis and three-vessel disease who are medically treated and those undergoing CABG.[16] Although these results were principally obtained in symptomatic patients, it seems reasonable to generalise them to asymptomatic patients following MI. In addition, despite their generally better prognosis, patients with double- and single-vessel disease are also likely to benefit from intervention when the disease affects a large volume of myocardium. It is carrying scientific rigorousness too far to restrict intervention to three-vessel and left main CHD patients. There is some evidence, for example, that proximal disease of the left anterior descending coronary artery (long known to practitioners of coronary angiography as the 'widow maker') is important,[17] yet such patients were consistently excluded from randomisation to surgery or medical therapy in the Coronary Artery Surgery Study (CASS).[18]

Therapeutics and risk factor modification

Skilled use of drug therapy probably contributes substantially to the benefits which accrue to the patient in a cardiac rehabilitation programme. This area of medical treatment also lends itself readily to relatively simple but powerful methods of audit. For example, a number of publications (eg Ref 19) demonstrate the lack of use of drugs with proven efficacy in the post-MI patient. This has been demonstrated for beta-blockers, and it is highly likely that many patients who could benefit from angiotensin-converting enzyme (ACE) inhibitors are simply not receiving this therapy. On the other hand, the uptake of drugs such as aspirin, which have almost universal applicability in patients with CHD, is probably much better.

The conditions amenable to recognition and treatment during cardiac follow-up include those listed in Table 1.

As discussed earlier, the appropriate therapy and reassessment of treatment efficacy within a rehabilitation programme are likely to

Table 1.
Some conditions amenable to recognition and treatment during cardiac follow-up.

- angina pectoris
- cardiac arrhythmias
- cardiac failure
- hyperlipidaemia and dyslipidaemia
- hypertension
- transient ischaemic attacks
- diabetes mellitus
- hyperuricaemia
- drug toxicity
- side effects

reduce long-term risk. Modification of risk factors, although difficult, is enhanced by multiple contacts between patient and therapist. This has been particularly well demonstrated for cigarette smoking, where regular reinforcement improves the efficacy of a smoking cessation programme.[20] Cigarette smoking is also a risk factor where there is clear evidence of benefit in patients who can stop smoking after an MI.[21]

Many patients with CHD will demonstrate a poor profile of plasma high- (HDL) and low-density lipoprotein (LDL) cholesterol and triglyceride — termed 'dyslipidaemia' to distinguish such patients from those with definite hyperlipidaemia. The latter usually have heterozygous familial hypercholesterolaemia, and there will be little controversy over the need for treatment. Moderate degrees of lipid abnormality may, however, carry an adverse prognosis in the patient with manifest CHD. There is increasing evidence that intervention with strict diet and/or lipid-lowering drugs can produce both atheroma regression and a reduction in long-term mortality. There is considerable potential for staff of a cardiac rehabilitation programme to impact on this risk factor.[22-24]

Other, newer risk factors continue to be described. For example, fibrinogen level is one of the most powerful predictors of risk in the post-MI patient, but it is not particularly influenced by any intervention other than smoking cessation and possibly fairly vigorous exercise.[25,26] Further research will reveal whether any drug-based approach would be of value in patients with high fibrinogen levels.

Programme management, efficacy and logistics

Management

A clinician involved with the cardiac rehabilitation programme who acts as the overall leader is important. Such a clinician will determine the attention paid to the various aspects of the programme according to the latest medical evidence and demonstrated therapeutic efficacy. For example, he may wish to set protocols for the measurement of and intervention by drug therapy for elevated plasma lipids. Problems are sometimes experienced by programme staff in implementing treatment or in investigation of programme participants, and it is important for the clinician to be able to act as a mediator when other medical staff need to be consulted about their patients. A variety of other staff contribute usefully to cardiac rehabilitation programmes but will not be further considered here. If the programme is run by a programme director or coordinator, this person needs regular contact with the lead clinician.

Efficacy

The efficacy of a cardiac rehabilitation programme can be determined by a number of measures which may also be considered as audit standards. A comprehensive list of these is found in the American Association of Cardiovascular and Pulmonary Rehabilitation (AACVPR) guidelines,[9] but a suggested list more appropriate for the UK is given in the appendix to this chapter.

Logistics

It is not possible to specify exactly the logistics of a cardiac rehabilitation programme. In the UK, the range of facilities is so wide, and the personnel involved with cardiac rehabilitation so varied, that the exact format by which a programme is run cannot be specified. Certain minimum standards, however, should be attained:

1. All staff involved with cardiac patients in rehabilitation should have basic life support training.

2. If no medical staff are present at any exercise session, at least one of the staff members present should be trained in advanced life support, of which the most important component is the ability to recognise and defibrillate ventricular fibrillation.

3. Exercise sessions unsupervised by medical staff should not

include 'high-risk' patients (in whatever way these are defined by the lead clinician and programme director).

4. Exercise sessions during Phase III of rehabilitation for low-risk patients (the organised outpatient training) should have rapid access to medical staff even if one is not present during the session.

5. Procedures for management of cardiac arrest should be rehearsed at intervals, and a record book kept.

6. Involvement of a resuscitation training officer in the programme is beneficial. High-risk patients should be offered the option of cardiopulmonary resuscitation training being given to their spouse, partner or close relatives.

7. Adequate record keeping of counselling and training sessions should be in place, also documentation of progress and other parameters, as dictated by research and audit protocols.

8. Equipment used should be registered under any asset registration schemes, and adequate and documented servicing and safety assessments made.

Conclusions

Medical input to cardiac rehabilitation is more than a sinecure. The best programmes, while enjoying the skills deployed by a wide variety of personnel, will always include a clinician with a complete overview of the needs of the cardiac patient. The links to many disciplines help in achieving the targets defined for the patients.

References

1. Oldridge NB, Guyatt GH, Fischer ME, Rimm AA. Cardiac rehabilitation after myocardial infarction. Combined experience of randomised clinical trials. *Journal of the American Medical Association* 1988;**260**:945–50.

2. O'Connor GT, Buring JE, Yusuf S, Goldhaber SZ, *et al.* An overview of randomised controlled trials of rehabilitation with exercise after myocardial infarction. *Circulation* 1989;**80**:234–44.

3. World Health Organisation. *Needs and action priorities in cardiac rehabilitation and secondary prevention in patients with CHD.* Geneva: WHO Regional Office for Europe, 1993.

4. The Multicentre Postinfarction Research Group. Risk stratification and survival after myocardial infarction. *New England Journal of Medicine* 1983;**309**:331–6.

5. Northridge DB, Hall RJC. Post-myocardial infarction exercise testing in the thrombolytic era. *Lancet* 1994;**343**:1175–6.

6. Campbell S, A'Hern R, Quigley P, Vincent R, *et al.* Identification of patients at low risk of dying after acute myocardial infarction by simple clinical and submaximal exercise test criteria. *European Heart Journal* 1988;**9**:938–47.

7. Gibson RS, Watson DD. Value of planar[201] Ti imaging in risk stratification of patients recovering from acute myocardial infarction. *Circulation* 1991;**84**(Suppl 1):1148–62.

8. Kulick DL, Rahimtoola SH. Risk stratification in survivors of acute myocardial infarction: routine cardiac catheterisation and angiography is a reasonable approach in most patients. *American Heart Journal* 1991;**121**:641–56.

9. American Association of Cardiovascular and Pulmonary Rehabilitation. *Guidelines for cardiac rehabilitation programs.* Champaign, IL: Human Kinetics, 1991.

10. Starling MR, Crawford MH, Kennedy GT, O'Rourke RA. Treadmill exercise tests predischarge and six weeks' post-myocardial infarction to detect abnormalities of known prognostic value. *Annals of Internal Medicine* 1981;**94**:849–53.

11. Mark DB, Shaw L, Harrell FE Jr, Hlatky MA, *et al.* Prognostic value of a treadmill exercise score in outpatients with suspected coronary artery disease. *New England Journal of Medicine* 1991;**325**:849–53.

12. Flapan AD. Management of patients after their first myocardial infarction. *British Medical Journal* 1994;**309**:1129–34.

13. Simoons ML, Vos J, Tijssen JGP, Vermeer F, *et al.* Long-term benefit of early thrombolytic therapy in patients with acute myocardial infarction: 5 year follow-up of a trial conducted by the Interuniversity Cardiology Institute of the Netherlands. *Journal of the American College of Cardiology* 1989;**14**:1609–15.

14. The TIMI Study Group. Comparison of invasive and conservative strategies after treatment with intravenous tissue plasminogen activator in acute myocardial infarction: results of the thrombolysis in myocardial infarction (TIMI) Phase II Trial. *New England Journal of Medicine* 1989;**320**:618–27.

15. The SWIFT (Should We Intervene Following Thrombolysis) Trial Study Group. The SWIFT trial of delayed elective intervention versus conservative treatment after thrombolysis with anistreplase in acute myocardial infarction. *British Medical Journal* 1991;**302**:555–60.

16. Yusuf S, Zucker D, Peduzzi, Fisher LD, *et al.* Effect of coronary bypass graft surgery on survival: overview of 10-year results from randomised trials by the Coronary Artery Bypass Graft Surgery Trialists Collaboration. *Lancet* 1994;**344**:563–70.

17. Schulman SP, Achuff SC, Griffith LS, Humphries JO, *et al.* Prognostic cardiac catheterization variables in survivors of acute myocardial infarction: a five year prospective study. *Journal of the American College of Cardiology* 1988;**11**:1164–72.

18. CASS principal investigators and their associates. Coronary Artery Surgery Study (CASS): a randomised trial of coronary artery bypass surgery. Survival data. *Circulation* 1983;**68**:939–50.

19. Whitford DL, Southern AJ. Audit of secondary prophylaxis after myocardial infarction. *British Medical Journal* 1994;**309**:1268–9.

20. Kottke TE, Battista RN, De Friese GH, Brekke ML. Attributes of successful smoking cessation interventions in medical practice. A meta-analysis of 39 controlled trials. *Journal of the American Medical Association* 1988;**259**:2883–9.

21. Aberg A, Bergstrand R, Johansson S, Ulvenstam G, *et al.* Cessation of smoking after myocardial infarction. Effects on mortality after 10 years. *British Heart Journal* 1983;**49**:416–22.

22. Schuler G, Hambrecht R, Schlierf G, Grunze M, *et al.* Myocardial perfusion and regression of coronary artery disease in patients on a regimen of intensive physical exercise and low fat diet. *Journal of the American College of Cardiology* 1992;**19**:34–42.

23. The Scandinavian Simvastatin Survival Study Group. Randomised trial of cholesterol lowering in 4444 patients with coronary heart disease: the Scandinavian Simvastatin Survival Study (4S). *Lancet* 1994;**344**:1383–9.

24. Heath GW, Ehsani AA, Hagberg JM, Hinderliter JM, Goldberg AP. Exercise training improves lipoprotein lipid profiles in patients with coronary artery disease. *American Heart Journal* 1983;**105**:889–95.

25. Meade TW, Ruddock V, Stirling Y, Chakrabarti R, Miller GJ. Fibrinolytic activity, clotting factors, and long term incidence of ischaemic heart disease in the Northwick Park Heart Study. *Lancet* 1993;**342**:1076–9.

26. Ferguson E, Bernier LL, Banta GR, Yu-Yahiro J, Schoomaker EB. Effects of exercise and conditioning on clotting and fibrinolytic activity in men. *Journal of Applied Physiology* 1987;**62**:1416–21.

Appendix

Audit standards

A post-infarction/CABG/PTCA counselling and advice programme should be in place in any district hospital which treats such patients. The percentage receiving formal counselling, even if not proceeding to a Phase III programme, should be recorded.

Risk stratification

Percentage of patients:

- undergoing post-MI exercise testing,
- undergoing post-MI perfusion imaging,

- receiving left ventricular function assessment by echo-cardiography or radionuclide ventriculography.

Further diagnostic testing and intervention

Percentage of patients receiving:

- diagnostic coronary arteriography,
- CABG,
- PTCA.

Interventions performed per patient-hours during the programme for:

- angina,
- dysrhythmia,
- heart failure,
- cardiac arrest.

Patients still experiencing angina at the end of the programme should be recorded, and also the percentage of such patients receiving diagnostic coronary arteriography.

Counselling or exercise sessions

Percentage of eligible:

- patients attending sessions,
- eligible female patients attending.

Median increment in fitness or effort tolerance by functional testing achieved in the programme. Frequency of minor and major orthopaedic complications per patient-hours of exercise.

Therapeutics and risk factor modification

Percentage of patients:

- taking aspirin,
- taking beta-blockers,
- taking ACE inhibitors,
- taking, or needing to use, sublingual nitrate therapy,

■ (and number) with systolic blood pressure above 160 mmHg or diastolic blood pressure below 90 mmHg at rest (eg at follow-up exercise test),

■ losing weight during the programme,

■ by pre-specified protocol (eg <75 years) whose plasma lipids (including HDL cholesterol) have been measured,

■ receiving follow-up lipid assessment,

■ showing a decrement in plasma LDL or an increase in plasma HDL cholesterol during the programme and follow-up,

■ showing a decrement in plasma triglyceride during follow-up,

■ receiving lipid-lowering medication,

■ recording smoking cessation, both short- and long-term (ideally, the self-reported figure should be compared with an objective measure such as exhaled carbon monoxide),

■ with psychosocial dysfunction or clinical depression (in programmes where this can be assessed).

The frequency of lipid assessment in relatives (particularly where high lipid levels appear to be the only risk factor for CHD).

3 The psychological component

Bob Lewin

Professor of Rehabilitation, School of Health, University of Hull

The goals of cardiac rehabilitation are to help the patient achieve the best possible quality of life and functional level, and to reduce morbidity and mortality through secondary prevention. Psychological factors are of major importance in achieving these aims for the following reasons:

- For most patients the main obstacles to recovering an acceptable quality of life are psychological and social, not physical.[1]

- Numerous studies have shown that the self-report of chest pain and disability,[2,3] the success of medical[4] and surgical treatment,[5] the use of medical resources post-myocardial infarction (MI),[6] and return to work[7] are related to scores measuring features such as anxiety, depression, cardiac misconceptions, hypochondriasis, anger and sleep disturbance, but *not* to disease measures.

- What the patient and his or her partner believe about the causes and course of coronary heart disease (CHD) is a major factor in determining their emotional and practical response to CHD, including adherence to medical treatment and any recommended lifestyle changes.[8]

- There is increasing evidence that psychological distress following MI is an independent risk factor for early mortality.[9–13]

The psychological goals

The main psychological goals of cardiac rehabilitation are:

1. To improve quality of life:

   - through the identification and treatment of psychological distress and psychiatric illness, and

   - by restoring confidence, thereby enabling patients to return to a full and active life.

2. To aid secondary prevention by:

    ■   helping patients initiate and maintain lifestyle changes, and

    ■   reducing psychological distress — there is some evidence from randomised intervention trials that this may also reduce mortality.[14]

The psychological sequelae of coronary heart disease

Post-MI adjustment has been well researched. Less is known about cardiac surgery patients who appear to manifest similar problems of adjustment, albeit with a lower incidence, and less still about transplant patients. Little is known about the psychological rehabilitation of patients with heart failure and angina, paediatric cardiac patients, patients with implanted cardioverter defibrillators, and those in the terminal stages of illness.

Adjustment to myocardial infarction or diagnosis of coronary heart disease

In most 'natural' disasters, the exposure to danger is time-limited, can be viewed as 'bad luck', and unlikely to be experienced again. Sustaining an MI or receiving the diagnosis of heart disease is equally frightening, but qualitatively different because:

■   to the lay mind, it implies a perpetual and largely inescapable risk of sudden or premature death;

■   it is often seen as the patient's own fault;

■   the factors that the patient believe responsible are often perceived as inherent to his or her character or life circumstances, and therefore impossible to change — lifestyle changes may be demanded that he or she fears cannot be maintained;

■   the diagnosis may also carry a significant threat to the financial and material well-being of the patient and his or her family.

Transplant patients

Transplant patients have particularly high levels of psychological distress. In one survey, up to 52% were regarded as psychologically distressed.[15] They have many of the same fears as other patients with CHD who are awaiting surgery, but differ in some aspects:

- psychiatric screening for selection is carried out by most centres, but there is little agreement about criteria or assessment methods;

- uncertainty about a donor increases anxiety, and it has been recommended that all such patients need psychological and social support during this waiting time;

- they are more prone to post-surgery delirium than other cardiac surgery patients, with reported incidence rates of 18–34%;

- anxiety may increase after surgery, and some authors have commented on the problems of adjustment to 'owning' a cadaver organ.[15]

The course of adjustment in hospital

Most patients with a suspected MI are clinically anxious on admission to hospital. The anxiety generally remits as the patient realises that he or she has survived the immediate crisis, but often rises again at the time of discharge home. In hospital, as many as 60% of patients may be anxious, half of whom may also be suffering from minor levels of depression. This distress is often deliberately hidden from the staff and other patients. Patients remaining without a diagnosis of MI are often more anxious than those who have had an infarct confirmed.[16] Following surgery, approximately 60% of patients report some psychological symptoms, the most common being increased anxiety, irritability, depression and confusion.[17] These symptoms usually remit over a few weeks. About 12–20% of patients are sceptical about having had a heart attack or their need for ongoing treatment, while others flatly contradict the physician's diagnosis.[18] An extreme form of denial has also occasionally been described in which the recently discharged patient explicitly tests himself against his 'fate' by indulging in strenuous activity or saturnalism excess shortly after the event,[19,20] although it is not recorded whether this has ever led to fatal consequences.

The course of adjustment following discharge

A reduction in mood, 'home coming depression', is so common as to be regarded as a normal part of the recovery process. In the majority of patients, unless there are further acute events, anxiety and depression slowly remit over the next few weeks, sometimes rising again at six weeks when return to work is imminent.[21]

Long-term psychological outcomes

For the sake of this discussion, three long-term outcomes may be described:

1. An improved quality of life.

2. Long-term psychological/psychiatric illness.

3. One or more aspect of quality of life deleteriously affected without (necessarily) a diagnosable psychological illness.

Improved quality of life

Following an MI, as many as 30% of patients regard their quality of life as equal or superior to that pre-infarct. The reasons given include:

- improving intimacy in relationships,

- increased joy in being alive,

- a re-evaluation of ambitions and the value of their relationships, and

- increased feeling of well-being through adopting a more healthy lifestyle.[22]

Continuing psychological illness

- A clinically significant degree of anxiety or depression is demonstrated by 15–30% of post-MI patients and 14–18% of post-coronary artery bypass patients which, if untreated, does not remit.

- There is little spontaneous change after the first months post-MI. Stern *et al*[23] found 70% of patients reporting depression at six weeks, and 67% of those anxious at three months were depressed or anxious at the one-year follow-up.

- The incidence of major depressive illness is low (10–15%), but significantly higher than in the general population.

- It is probable that as many as 50% of the individuals who manifest a major psychiatric illness post-MI have had a pre-existing psychiatric problem.[24]

- Major depressive illness is unlikely to remit unless treated.

- The incidence of psychotic illness appears to be very low and no more common than in the general population.

■ A small number of patients will succumb to a restricted and fearful lifestyle that has been labelled in many different ways over the years (eg 'cardiac neurosis', 'neurocirculatory asthenia', 'effort syndrome'). These patients are currently described as demonstrating 'undue illness behaviour'. They are typified by high levels of anxiety, increasing physical deconditioning due to the avoidance of exercise, a hopeless and dependent attitude, and an almost obsessional preoccupation with physical symptoms and the details of their medical history.[25] They are frequently hospitalised for further, usually fruitless, investigations.

■ Partners and other family members are often more psychologically disturbed than the patient, which may have an important influence on the patient's own anxiety and long-term outcome.[26,27]

Reduced quality of life

It has been claimed that as many as 40–60% of patients have some long-term reduction in their quality of life, mainly as the result of psychological factors.[28] This group may be subdivided into two main categories:

■ those who manifest a global reduction in confidence, and

■ those in whom only a discrete area of life has been affected (eg sexual adjustment or premature and unwanted retirement).

Most of the first group appear well to others, and will confirm this on casual enquiry, but family and friends usually say that 'they are not their old selves'. When directly questioned, many patients will admit to a constant painful awareness that they are now 'a heart patient'.

Common problems reducing quality of life in patients with coronary heart disease

Perception of health

Sustaining an MI has a powerful effect on the perception of health. In one cohort, 67% of the patients retrospectively rated their pre-infarct health as 'high'. Following discharge from hospital, this percentage had sunk to 21%, and at 3–5 years post-MI only 42% regarded themselves as having recovered their health.[29] These beliefs naturally predispose patients to an increased and often unnecessary use of health services.

Activity

The most common reaction of patients after an MI is to fear and deliberately avoid activity. Normal or explicable feelings of fatigue or minor symptoms tend to be interpreted as relating to the heart, often leading to a reduction in social and physical activity and further preoccupation with symptoms.[30] Reduced activity automatically leads to physical deconditioning, producing more fatigue and therefore further anxiety, and patients often become trapped in a downward spiral of increasing disability. A survey by Finlayson and McEwen[31] found that at one and four years 30% and 50%, respectively, of their sample of post-MI patients reported a reduction in social and leisure activities. Croog and Levine[32] found that 70% of an American group reported being less active 12 months after their infarct.

Return to work

Reports of return to work following MI vary between 40% and 92%. Cultural variations in welfare benefits explain part of this variation. Another reason is the sampling point chosen: many patients return to work, but retire prematurely. Mayou[33] reported that 90% of a cohort returned to work, but one year later only 70% were still in work. Several studies have found that in approximately 50% of cases the primary reasons for failure to return to work are psychological: depression, overprotection by the family, fear of harm, and attribution of the MI to stress at work.[5,34] Once back at work, some patients deliberately reduce their activity levels, believe that their health has damaged their work capacity, and report reduced earnings and greater work-related stress.[35]

Return to work following bypass is equally disappointing. It is strongly influenced by the time off work prior to the operation. An early study found that patients off work for longer than six months had a 50% chance of permanent invalidism. The best predictor of return to work is the patient's expectation prior to surgery of returning.[36]

Relationships

Good marriages, in common with other forms of social support, have been recorded as having a 'buffering effect', reducing distress and improving outcome, but previously poor relationships (20% of male American patients blamed the heart attack on their wives) are often further jeopardised by a reduction in communication. A dramatic increase in irritability has been widely reported as a source of friction in relationships. This is more commonly reported in male patients, with spouses often feeling that dealing with the patient is like 'walking on eggshells' or 'living with a volcano'. It is reported that the wives of high 'deniers', who continue to indulge in risk behaviour are at particular risk of psychological disturbance.

Sexual activity

In the first months of recovery 30–50% of post-MI patients are afraid of resuming sex, usually because of the common misconception that orgasm is particularly likely to cause infarction. Long-term sexual problems of a psychogenic nature have been reported in 20–58% of cardiac patients. Post-MI patients are particularly affected: about 15% report increased satisfaction, 25% are unaffected, 25% never resume sexual activity, with the remainder experiencing reduced frequency and/or pleasure.[36] Partners share the same worries, and their fear is often the major factor in reduced sexual activity and enjoyment.[37]

Anxiety and depression in partners

Following MI, partners are often more distressed than the patients. A study of 52 spouses revealed that 26% of those who were anxious or depressed felt guilty, believing that their own actions might have caused the problem. In several cases, this belief had been directly fostered by the patient. There appear to be two other major causes of distress:

- A fear of provoking another infarct by doing or saying something that might cause the patient worry or annoyance.

- At the time of the infarct, the spouse took over all the patient's familial tasks and responsibilities, expecting this to be temporary, but months later the patient was showing no sign of resuming his or her share of the work, thus causing the healthy partner to feel stressed and/or resentful.

The main predictors of rehabilitation outcome

It has repeatedly been shown that there is no correlation between the severity of infarction and the degree of psychological disturbance in MI patients. Some well established correlates of poor rehabilitation outcome are:

- *Anxiety and depression,* especially with a previous history.

- The number of *cardiac misconceptions* held by the patient.[7] Even after cardiac education classes about risk factors, approximately 80% of post-MI patients blame stress, worry or overwork as the primary reason for their illness. They view the heart as 'worn out', and fear and avoid activity that they think will further deplete their energy reserves. These damaging beliefs are often reinforced by the media, friends and family, and sometimes by lifestyle advice received from medical care staff. Bypass and angina patients have additional misconceptions, for example, that 'strain' could 'dislodge the graft', and that an episode of angina is a 'mini heart attack'.

- *Poor communication* from clinical staff may account for as much as 20% of unwarranted invalidism. Particular problems are overguarded statements about the patient's prognosis, and vague advice such as 'just be sensible', or statements such as 'part of your heart is dead' or 'your arteries are blocked up'.[34]

- *Lower educational level and lower social class* are predictors, probably both because of their relationship with the factors above, and because of a greater threat to employment and its relationship to social deprivation which increases morbidity and mortality in all disease states.[38]

- Despite there being no relationship between *perceived health status* and the severity of the MI, the former is related to a number of measures of recovery including return to work, 'involvement with symptoms', use of health resources, and anxiety and depression.[4]

- *Perceived stress and social isolation.*

- *Personality variables,* for example, hypochondriasis, neuroticism, and a 'passive fearful coping style'.

The integration of cardiac rehabilitation with routine medical care

Almost all CHD patients and their families have to make a large psychological adjustment. Scant attention is paid to this in routine medical care, which centres around ensuring survival, physical

investigations, and medical and surgical treatment. Poor psychological adjustment can often be traced to inadequate attention
being paid to the patient's psychological needs. The provision of a
successful rehabilitation service will depend upon these needs being
met as part of the routine medical and nursing care to which the
patient is exposed, both in hospital and following discharge.

The hospital phase

There is a consensus that cardiac rehabilitation should begin at the
time of diagnosis of CHD, or as soon as possible following admission
with an acute event.[39]

Counselling

Counselling is a portmanteau expression covering a wide range of
styles, theoretical beliefs and aims. The majority of patients do not
need, or want,[40] counselling for 'emotional support'. Indeed, there
is evidence that such support does not improve outcome over that
achieved by advice and relaxation supplied on audio tape.[41]
However, counselling as a two-way process of exploring and correcting cardiac misconceptions, and of increasing information and
coping skills *is* an essential part of the rehabilitation process. As
soon as possible after the acute event or diagnosis all patients and,
where possible, their partners should receive counselling, with the
following aims:

- To correct the common *misconceptions* about the causes of CHD,
  its prognosis, the healing properties of bed-rest, the dangers of
  sex, and the contribution to MI of stress, worry and overwork.
  Where time is limited, the eradication of these harmful negative
  misconceptions should have the first priority.

- It is important to provide a *'cause'* whenever possible; this
  should be the patient's own set of risk factors, and the ability
  to control them should be emphasised.

- All patients should be given detailed, practical and *encouraging*
  information and advice about the secondary prevention
  measures they can take for themselves. Academic reserva-
  tions, qualifications and complications should be avoided —
  without conveying untruths — because anxious patients are
  liable to fasten on to these as further bad news. Particular care
  should be taken to avoid unintentionally reinforcing cardiac
  misconceptions about stress.

- Some people are not aware of the *lifestyle factors* that lead to CHD, so all patients and their families should be given information and advice, preferably backed up with written material. The advice should be realistic and practical (many patients are extremely poor), concrete, specify exactly what should be done (eg 'eat five portions of fresh fruit or vegetables every day' instead of 'try to eat more fruit'), and also take account of social and ethnic variation. For the reasons given above, naïve advice about avoiding 'stress' is likely to be harmful.

- Patients should be helped to develop an individualised and concrete *plan for recovery* to be carried out on discharge. The resumption of activity should proceed in a systematic stepwise progression. A formal method for achieving this can be taught to patients before they go home. Vague advice such as 'listen to your body' or 'do what you can manage' is unhelpful.

- Patients and their families should be warned about the *physical and psychological sequelae* that may become apparent for the first time on returning home. An explanation should be given that normalises these symptoms, and presents them as universal and part of the natural course of recovery following *any* potentially life-threatening event. The primary physical symptoms are unexpected weakness due to conditioning, breathlessness on exercise, and angina. Common psychological reactions to mention are low mood, including tearfulness, sleep disturbance, irritability, anxiety, acute awareness of minor somatic sensations or pains, and poor concentration and memory.

- *Delay in seeking help* in MI may account for 50% of out-of-hospital deaths, and patients having a reinfarction delay for as long as those with a first MI. This delay is extended when other people are present. Patients and spouses should be given written advice and a plan to follow if they experience the symptoms of MI.

- Partners should be advised to alter the *family routines* as little as possible, except for lifestyle changes such as smoking or diet which should begin immediately.

- Tactful *advice* must be given about not overprotecting the patient or, in a few cases, from expecting her (it is usually female patients) to resume doing all the housework immediately. The understanding of this advice, by both patient and partner, should be checked by asking them to summarise it during and at the end of each session.

- Patients have their own *beliefs about CHD* which are markedly different from the 'medical model'. There is evidence that it is ineffective simply to tell patients what to believe without taking this difference into account.[42] All staff coming in contact with patients should be trained to provide such counselling, and adequate time should be allowed for this. Every member of the clinical team coming in contact with the patient and his or her family should be aware of the content of this counselling and reinforce the information given to the patient (who may deliberately check to see if other members of staff agree).

- It is helpful to provide *written or tape-recorded advice* (the interview itself can be taped) because 50% of verbal advice given in a five-minute consultation is forgotten within a further five minutes.[43]

- Evidence that this approach is worthwhile comes from two randomised controlled trials:

  - One study[44] involved the patient and his or her partner in four half-hour sessions of counselling similar to that described above, commencing within 24 hours of admission. This intervention reduced anxiety and depression by 50%, and provided significant improvements in a number of other rehabilitative outcomes in patient and partner.

  - Similar improvements were seen with a written and tape-based, self-help rehabilitation programme.[45] This was based on the same principles of correcting cardiac misconceptions and providing a planned return to activity. It was introduced to the patient in a half-hour structured interview three days post-MI by a trained nurse facilitator who also provided brief counselling and encouragement on three further occasions over the next six weeks.

Dealing with denial

Some authorities believe denial to be predictive of a good outcome, some see it as a mechanism concealing extreme fear, and others as the result of ignorance. If it leads to medical non-compliance, it may be a problem; otherwise, the evidence suggests that moderate levels of denial in a well informed patient may be a helpful short-term coping strategy and should not be officiously disturbed.

Exercise

In the majority of cases, a simple, very low level exercise programme can begin on the ward and be continued once the patient gets home.

Relaxation training

Many patients value a relaxation tape in the coronary care unit (CCU), step-down or general ward. Patients can be given the tape to continue practising at home. A few patients are made *more* anxious by relaxation, and nursing staff should be aware of how to deal with this problem.

Hase and Douglas[46] demonstrated both a significant reduction in anxiety and a number of longer-term benefits for patients given a tape to listen to in the CCU. For example, at the four-month follow-up, the experimental group claimed to be walking further than the control group (6.7 km per week vs 2.7 km per week), they reported significantly fewer episodes of chest pain (0.40 vs 2.13 per week) and there was a 50% reduction in the number of patients who reported 'psychological problems' (10 vs 25).

Guzzetta[47] found significantly lower mean heart rates and higher peripheral temperatures in a group in the CCU administered a relaxation tape than in a control group. When patients were asked how helpful the sessions were in helping them to relax, 92% said 'extremely helpful' and 77% said they would continue to practise these techniques following discharge from the CCU.

Helpline

Anxiety typically rises at discharge, and most patients appreciate being given a telephone number to call if they have any medical concerns; this should be available over 24 hours, and the CCU number is often the most appropriate. Experience shows that this facility is rarely abused by patients.

Post-discharge

Early convalescence

Many patients are back at home before they have fully taken in what has happened to them. At home, they are surrounded by family, friends and neighbours who may advise them to take prolonged rest, give up work and make other precipitate, unnecessary and unhelpful adaptations. Unfortunately, for organisational reasons, many patients do not have an exercise tolerance test or join a rehabilitation programme for as long as 10 weeks' post-discharge. Ideally, rehabilitation should continue seamlessly after discharge as it is important that encouragement towards mobilisation and lifestyle changes begun in hospital should continue in the community. It is essential that patients do not wait to resume their life until their 'check-up' or commencing a rehabilitation programme.

In the great majority of cases, a simple home-based exercise programme, and/or daily programme of brisk walking, 'paced up' in a controlled manner, can be commenced from discharge and brings similar physiological benefits as hospital-based exercise programmes.[45,48,49]

At follow-up clinics, the advice about secondary prevention and resumption of the normal activities of daily living should be stressed, enquired about and encouraged.

It is important that advice given in the community does not conflict with the advice given by the secondary care team. In particular, patients who have been advised to avoid prolonged rest on returning home are sometimes told to rest by their general practitioner (GP). It would be useful if the advice given in hospital could be communicated to the GP in the discharge letter.

Rehabilitation programme

The majority of rehabilitation programmes centre around group exercise classes.[50] One difficulty with this is that patients who are unable, or do not want, to exercise may be excluded or exclude themselves. It has often been suggested that a superior option would be for programmes to be based on a 'menu system', whereby the patients' needs are assessed and they are offered only those elements of cardiac rehabilitation they require. The other elements accepted as useful are:

- lifestyle changes (secondary prevention),
- relaxation classes,
- stress management classes, and
- individual treatment from a psychologist or liaison psychiatrist for patients identified as being particularly distressed.[51]

For example, a patient who was previously physically active, is now walking several miles a day, has stopped smoking and changed his diet, but is delaying a return to work because he feels anxious about its stressful nature, may only require to attend a psychologist or a stress management class. On the other hand, a patient who has never exercised, has failed to alter risk behaviour and is anxious, will require all the elements of the programme. If patients have received the inpatient and post-discharge support described above, the number requiring a further extensive rehabilitation programme will be minimised.

Psychological factors in exercise training

Controlled trials have almost universally reported that exercise and advice alone do not produce long-term improvements in overall psychosocial adjustment in post-MI or surgery patients,[52–59] neither do they appear to improve return to work rates.[6] This was a great disappointment and something of a mystery to the pioneers of cardiac rehabilitation who assumed that as patients experienced a return of functional ability they would make use of it, and that this would restore confidence.[60] Anxious patients are known not to regard functional ability as related to health status. The major predictors of return to work are perceived health status, the number of cardiac misconceptions, anxiety, depression, and various other psychosocial variables. Unfortunately, despite this, many rehabilitation programmes continue to rely on increasing patients' fitness level as the main method for restoring lost confidence and quality of life. However, increasing (and then maintaining) fitness can significantly improve symptoms such as angina and fatigue.[61–62]

There is evidence that attending exercise classes has a small effect on anxiety and depression — but not sufficient to be clinically useful — nor does the degree of relief appear to be related to the degree of increase of aerobic fitness. The effects may be produced through increased feelings of personal control over illness.[63] In patients with significantly raised anxiety or depression, effects are similarly small and are lost over 12 months.

Non-compliance is a major problem in fitness training. For example, it has been reported that in some centres as many as 50% of patients drop out before the end of an exercise programme, and follow-up studies have reported that as few as 30% may still be exercising one year later.[64] Strategies to improve long-term compliance and the factors that contribute to drop-out have been studied,[65] but the findings appear to be largely ignored. Briefly, compliance is increased where exercise is regular (ie daily rather than weekly), close at hand, built into daily living (eg walking to work), perceived as enjoyable — or at least not aversive — and does not involve financial or time costs.

Patients with particularly 'heavy' jobs are more likely to develop the confidence to return to work if they can take part in 'work hardening' exercises — the more similar the tasks are to the actual tasks demanded by the job the better. Such exercise should be combined with explicit counselling for return to work.

Counselling

The importance of reversing the cardiac misconceptions has already been addressed. Ideally, this began in hospital, and it is important that patients (and their partners) who continue to hold these beliefs have further counselling post-discharge. Patients should be helped to recommence those activities of which they are fearful in small steps practised daily or as regularly as possible; in this way, the fear usually subsides. Partners who are afraid to let the patient out of their sight or frequently wake the patient during the night to see if he is still alive can have their anxiety reduced in a similar way.

Relaxation

Most multidisciplinary rehabilitation programmes provide relaxation classes. The few studies that have been conducted suggest they may be of value. Relaxation should be taught as a coping technique for use in real-life situations, and rapidly move on from being taught lying down listening to an instructor to self-applied techniques and rapid relaxation that can be used in any situation.

Van Dixhoorn *et al*[66] found that the addition of breathing and relaxation training to a post-MI exercise programme improved training success by 50%, as well as significantly reducing ST segment abnormalities. Follow-up at 2–3 years revealed that patients who received both treatments had significantly fewer cardiac events (17% vs 37%) than those who had undergone exercise training alone.[67]

A Medical Research Council trial of relaxation training in high-risk (moderately hypertensive) patients demonstrated useful reduction in blood pressure and fewer acute cardiac events over the following four years,[68] suggesting that it may have a role in secondary prevention.

Stress management training

As with counselling, the term 'stress management' has no fixed meaning and no recognised training or qualification. It usually includes relaxation training with additional techniques, but these vary widely and, at worst, it may consist of little more than a talk and one or more complementary therapies. The rationale for its use in rehabilitation is to reduce distress by teaching patients to gain control over situations that lead to unpleasantly high levels of stress response (autonomic arousal). It should include an assessment of such situations, teach patients new ways of coping, such as relaxation, distraction or positive self-talk, and then involve them in practising these techniques in real-life situations. In the majority of cases, the stress response will be triggered by some perceived threat (which is usually unrealistically alarming). Patients need to be taught methods for identifying these thoughts and how to evaluate their validity. They should also be helped to recognise the contribution that their own and other people's behaviour makes to their stress, and learn time management, assertiveness and other skills to reduce these problems.

Patients who notice an increase of symptoms such as angina or breathlessness when 'stressed' or who are particularly afraid of stress producing sudden death, may benefit from stress management classes. In suggesting these, care must be taken not to reinforce the patients' cardiac misconceptions and anxiety about the dangers of 'stress'.

A controlled comparison between stress management and relaxation alone[69] produced a significant improvement in a number of rehabilitative end-points in both treated groups. At six months, the former group had fewer cardiac complications (10% vs 31%) than those given only relaxation. In another controlled trial,[14] stress management was not taught, but patients were monitored for a rise in emotional distress using a telephone questionnaire administered monthly; if the patient exhibited an elevated score, a nurse was sent to the patient to solve the underlying problem. Distress was reduced, and the death rate halved in the year after MI.

Secondary prevention

There is evidence that some changes in lifestyle can bring about worthwhile secondary prevention.[51] One trial[70] has shown that sufficiently comprehensive lifestyle changes can halt or even bring about a regression of CHD. Unfortunately though, 50% of the patients approached refused to enter the trial. Also, an important element in the trial was the provision of extensive ongoing social support that would be difficult to provide in the National Health Service.

Adopting secondary prevention measures can significantly aid psychological recovery by increasing the patient's belief in his or her ability to control the disease process. For this reason alone, clinical staff should take a firm, optimistic and encouraging stance on all forms of helpful behaviour change. The naïve view that frightening patients increases compliance with these changes has been disproved on numerous occasions (eg Ref 43). It is far better to motivate patients through stressing the positive aspects of such changes, without minimising the difficulties.

The main technique that is used by most rehabilitation programmes to bring about secondary prevention is talks from health care staff. There is evidence that educational sessions can increase the patients' knowledge about heart disease, encourage some short-term changes in health behaviours, and may help to reduce some negative psychosocial consequences in the year after MI. However, in most individuals, education classes do not produce changes in smoking,[71] diet,[72] compliance with exercise advice[64,73] or reduce clinical levels of psychological disturbance.[74,75] The necessity to provide information for those who need it has been mentioned, but the value of most didactic health-change 'talks' is limited, and there is poor compliance with advice one year after an acute event.[75]

There is evidence that current information-giving techniques are inadequate, often not complied with, and retention of information is not checked. Many patients put more store on the information given to them by family and friends.[76] Advice on the resumption of sex is largely ignored and, when information is given, it is often inaccurate.[77]

Anxious patients often benefit from an explanation of the associated symptoms (eg raised pulse rate, sudden feelings of weakness, nausea) in terms of adrenaline and the 'fight or flight' mechanism. Without this understanding, they tend to relate these symptoms to their cardiac condition, which often serves to increase symptoms further, sometimes resulting in acute anxiety and, in some individuals, unnecessary emergency admission.

Ideally, partners should be equally involved in the educational aspects of the rehabilitation process, although they may have somewhat different needs.[78]

Cognitive behavioural treatment for lifestyle changes

Cognitive behavioural treatment (CBT) may be a more promising method for producing lasting changes in lifestyle. It encourages patients to examine the beliefs, motivations and environmental factors that maintain their unwanted behaviour. Most importantly, it involves them in systematically practising the new behaviours. Important elements of CBT are checking progress, providing feedback about reduced risk, solving problems that have arisen, and providing encouragement to continue. The process must be continued over months; it requires specially trained medical staff, and is expensive in time and resources. Approximately 50% of patients will make the necessary changes without help, so it is important to screen for the patients who require assistance and not to provide such help universally.

Exercise programmes that have incorporated CBT methods have shown worthwhile gains in long-term compliance,[64] as have programmes aimed at maintaining weight loss[79] and smoking cessation.[80]

A controlled trial of a CBT-based programme for cardiac risk factor reduction in a high-risk but well population produced a 41% reduction in the overall CHD risk one year later.[81]

The role of the psychologist or liaison psychiatrist

During the inpatient phase the main role of the psychologist or liaison psychiatrist is to provide treatment for the relatively small number of patients who have acute mental health problems or present management problems. Patients with clinical levels of anxiety or depression should be treated by health care staff with mental health training at postgraduate level (ie a clinical psychologist or psychiatrist). An interest in counselling or attendance at training courses is not a sufficient qualification for the diagnosis and treatment of psychological illness. A psychiatrically trained nurse who is supervised as part of a mental health team may also be a suitable person to see these patients. A psychologist may be helpful in designing relevant assessment and audit procedures and in training staff in counselling skills, and may also be a useful member of a multidisciplinary rehabilitation team.

All acute centres and rehabilitation programmes will have psychologically distressed patients, and in designing services funding should be allocated to purchase treatment for them. Clinically significant levels of anxiety or depression that may benefit from treatment will be experienced by 10–18% of patients. A higher proportion of patients will show symptoms of reactive anxiety or depression, but in most cases the distress will be transitory and the counselling sessions described above, which should be conducted by a member of the clinical care team, should be sufficient.

Psychological assessment

Psychological distress

It is not possible to determine mental status by observation alone. Psychological distress should be screened for and measured using well validated questionnaires standardised for a medically ill population. Suitable questionnaires are:

- the Hospital Anxiety and Depression Scale,[82] and
- the General Health Questionnaire (12- or 30-item version).[83]

Both questionnaires are short, extensively validated, acceptable to the general population, can be administered by post or telephone, and are easy to score.

Psychological status in hospital is only moderately related to long-term outcome. Patients should also be screened at 6–12 weeks. Patients still markedly distressed at this time will require referral for psychological/psychiatric treatment if they are to improve.[84]

Cognitive dysfunction

Post-bypass patients suffer an excess of cognitive dysfunction. Lower levels of similar problems are found in post-MI patients, and both groups frequently complain of problems with memory and attention. In most cases, the later problems are related to anxiety. It can be useful to carry out a neuropsychological assessment in patients who are particularly worried about this and in those who might have suffered anoxia and have subsequently become mysteriously 'stuck' in their resumption of a normal life.

Other outcomes

The goals of rehabilitation are complex:

- a maximal quality of life and well-being,
- restored confidence and functional ability, and
- reduced illness behaviour.

Current quality of life assessments tend to be more suitable for research than for clinical practice. At present, there does not appear to be a suitable British measure for assessing these needs, comparing outcome between treatment methods and/or for conducting clinical audit.

References

1. Kallio V, Cay E. *Rehabilitation after myocardial infarction. The European experience.* Copenhagen: World Health Organisation, Regional Office for Europe, 1985.

2. Smith TW, Follick MJ, Korr KS. Anger, neuroticism, type A behaviour and the experience of angina. *British Journal of Medical Psychology* 1984;**57**:249–52.

3. Jenkins DC, Stanton B, Klien MD, *et al.* Correlates of angina pectoris amongst men awaiting coronary artery bypass surgery. *Psychosomatic Medicine* 1983;**45**:141–53.

4. Williams RB, Haney TH, McKinnis RA. Psychosocial and physical predictors of angina pain relief with medical management. *Psychosomatic Medicine* 1986;**48**:200–10.

5. Channer KS, O'Connor S, Britton S. Psychological status during recovery from an acute heart attack. *Journal of the Royal Society of Medicine* 1988;**11**:629–32.

6. Maeland JG, Havik OE. Use of health services after a myocardial infarction. *Scandinavian Journal of Social Medicine* 1989;**17**:93–102.

7. Danchin N, Goepfert PC. Exercise training, cardiac rehabilitation and return to work in patients with coronary artery disease. *European Heart Journal* 1988;**9**:43–6.

8. Maeland JG, Havik OE. After the myocardial infarction. A medical and psychological study with special emphasis on perceived illness. *Scandinavian Journal of Rehabilitation Medicine* 1989;**22**(Suppl):1–87.

9. Garrity TF, Klein RF. Emotional response and clinical severity as early determinants of six-month mortality after myocardial infarction. *Heart and Lung* 1975;**4**:730–7.

10. Ruberman W, Weinblatt E, Goldberg JD, Chaudhary BS. Psychosocial influences on mortality after myocardial infarction. *New England Journal of Medicine* 1984;**311**:552–9.

11. Carney RM, Rich MW, Freedland KE, Saini J. Major depressive disorder predicts cardiac events in patients with coronary artery disease. *Psychosomatic Medicine* 1988;**50**:627–33.

12. Brackett CD, Powell LH. Psychosocial and physiological predictors of sudden cardiac death after healing of acute myocardial infarction. *American Journal of Cardiology* 1988;**61**:979–83.

13. Frasure-Smith N. In-hospital symptoms of psychological stress as predictors of long-term outcome following acute myocardial infarction in men. *American Journal of Cardiology* 1991;**67**:121–7.

14. Frasure-Smith N, Prince R. Long-term follow-up of the ischaemic heart disease life stress monitoring program. *Psychosomatic Medicine* 1989;**51**:485–513.

15. Mai F. Psychiatric aspects of heart transplantation. *British Journal of Psychiatry* 1993;**163**:285–92.

16. Cay EL, Vetter N, Philip A, Dugard P. Psychological status during recovery from an acute heart attack. *Journal of Psychosomatic Research* 1972;**16**:425–35.

17. Soloff PH. Medically and surgically treated coronary patients in cardio-vascular rehabilitation — a comparative study. *International Journal of Psychiatry in Medicine* 1979;**9**:93–106.

18. Almeida D, Wenger NK. Emotional responses of patients with acute myocardial infarction to their disease. *Cardiology* 1982;**69**:303–9.

19. Gulledge AD. Psychological aftermaths of myocardial infarction. In: Gentry WD, Williams RB (eds). *Psychological aspects of myocardial infarction.* St Louis, MI: CV Mosby, 1979:113–30.

20. Soloff PH. Denial and rehabilitation of the postinfarction patient. *International Journal of Psychiatry in Medicine* 1978;**8**:125–32.

21. Thompson DR, Webster RA, Cordle CJ, Sutton TW. Specific sources of anxiety in male patients with first myocardial infarction. *British Journal of Medical Psychology* 1987;**60**:343–8.

22. Laerum E, Johnsen N, Smith P, Larsen S. Myocardial infarction may induce positive changes in lifestyle and in the quality of life. *Scandinavian Journal of Primary Health Care* 1988;**6**:67–71.

23. Stern MJ, Pascal L, McLoone JB. Psychosocial adaptation following an acute myocardial infarction. *Journal of Chronic Diseases* 1976;**29**:513–26.

24. Lloyd GG, Cawley RH. Distress or illness? A study of psychological symptoms after myocardial infarction. *British Journal of Psychiatry* 1993;**142**:120–5.

25. Julian DG. *Cardiology,* 6th edn. London: Baillière Tindall, 1992.

26. Doerr BC, Jones JW. Effects of family preparation on the state anxiety level of the CCU patient. *Nursing Research* 1979;**28**:315–6.

27. Cay EL. Psychological problems in patients after a myocardial infarction. *Advances in Cardiology* 1982;**22**:108–12.

28. Wiklund I, Sanne H, Elmfeldt D, Vedin A, Wilhelmsson C. Emotional reaction, health preoccupation and sexual activity two months after a myocardial infarction. *Scandinavian Journal of Rehabilitation Medicine* 1984;**16**:47–56.

29. Maeland JG, Havik OE. Self-assessment of health before and after a myocardial infarction. *Social Science and Medicine* 1988;**27**:297–305.

30. Wiklund I, Sanne H, Vedin A, Wilhelmsson C. Psychosocial outcome one year after a first myocardial infarction. *Journal of Psychosomatic Research* 1984;**28**:309–21.

31. Finlayson A, McEwen J. *Coronary heart disease and patterns of living.* London: Croom Helm, 1977.

32. Croog SH, Levine S. *The heart patient recovers.* New York: Human Science Press, 1977.

33. Mayou R. The course and determinants of reactions to myocardial infarction. *British Journal of Psychiatry* 1979;**134**:588–94.

34. Wynn A. Unwarranted emotional distress in men with ischaemic heart disease. *Medical Journal of Australia* 1967;**2**:847–51.

35. Hinora S. Psychological aspects in the rehabilitation of coronary heart disease. *Scandinavian Journal of Rehabilitation Medicine* 1970;**12**:53–9.

36. Sanne H, Wenger NK. Sexual function/dysfunction and rehabilitative counselling. In: *Psychology and social aspects of coronary heart disease: information for the clinician.* CT: International Society and Federation of Cardiology, Le Jacq Communications Inc, 1988:48–54.

37. Cooper AJ. Myocardial infarction and advice on sexual activity. *Practitioner* 1985;**229**:575–9.

38. Davey Smith G, Bartley M, Blane D. The Black Report on socio-economic inequalities in health 10 years on. *British Medical Journal* 1990;**301**:373–7.

39. World Health Organisation. *Needs and action priorities in cardiac rehabilitation and secondary prevention in patients with CHD.* Geneva: WHO Regional Office for Europe, 1993.

40. Orzeck SA, Staniloff HP. Comparison of patients' and spouses' needs during the posthospital convalescence phase of a myocardial infarction. *Journal of Cardiopulmonary Rehabilitation* 1987;**7**:59–67.

41. Oldenberg B, Perkins RJ. Controlled trial of psychological intervention in myocardial infarction. *Journal of Consulting and Clinical Psychology* 1985;**53**:852–9.

42. Fielding R. Patients' beliefs regarding the causes of myocardial infarction: implications for information-giving and compliance. *Patient Education and Counseling* 1987;**9**:121–34.

43. Ley P. Psychological studies of doctor-patient communication. In: Rachman S (ed). *Contributions to medical psychology.* Oxford: Pergamon, 1977:9–42.

44. Thompson DR. *Counselling the coronary patient and partner.* London: Scutari, 1990.

45. Lewin B, Robertson IH, Cay EL, Irving JB, *et al.* Effects of self-help post-myocardial infarction rehabilitation on psychological adjustment and use of health services. *Lancet* 1992;**339**:1036–40.

46. Hase S, Douglas A. Effects of relaxation training on recovery from myocardial infarction. *Australian Journal of Advanced Nursing* 1987;**5**:18–26.

47. Guzzetta CE. Effects of relaxation and music therapy on patients in a coronary care unit with presumed acute myocardial infarction. *Heart and Lung* 1989;**18**:609–16.

48. DeBusk R, Haskell W, Miller N, Berra K, Taylor CB. Medically directed at-home rehabilitation soon after uncomplicated myocardial infarction: a new model for patient care. *American Journal of Cardiology* 1985;**55**:251–7.

49. Goble AJ, Hare DL, MacDonald PS, Oliver RG, *et al.* Effects of early pro-grammes of high and low intensity exercise on physical performance after transmural acute myocardial infarction. *British Heart Journal* 1991;**65**:126–31.

50. Horgan J, Bethell H, Carson P, Davidson C, *et al.* Working party report on cardiac rehabilitation. *British Heart Journal* 1992;**67**:412–8.

51. World Health Organisation. *Cardiac rehabilitation and secondary prevention: long term care for patients with ischaemic heart disease.* Briefing letter. Copenhagen: WHO Regional Office for Europe, 1993.

52. Naughton J, Balke B, Poarch A. Modified work capacity studies in individuals with and without coronary artery disease. *Journal of Sports Medicine and Physical Fitness* 1964;**4**:208–12.

53. Plavsic C, Turkulin K, Perman Z, Steinnes S, *et al.* The results of exercise therapy in coronary prone individuals and coronary patients. *Journal of Italian Cardiology* 1976;**6**:422–32.

54. Mayou R, MacMahon D, Sleight P, Florencio MJ. Early rehabilitation after myocardial infarction. *Lancet* 1981;**ii**:1399–401.

55. Stern MJ, Cleary P. The National Exercise and Heart Disease Project: long term psychosocial outcome. *Archives of Internal Medicine* 1982;**142**:1093–7.

56. Greenland P, Chu JS. Efficacy of cardiac services with emphasis on patients after myocardial infarction. *Annals of Internal Medicine* 1988;**109**:650–3.

57. Lipkin DP. Is cardiac rehabilitation necessary? *British Heart Journal* 1991;**65**:237–8.

58. Oldridge NB, Guyatt G, Jones N, Crowe J, *et al.* Effects on quality of life with comprehensive rehabilitation after acute myocardial infarction. *American Journal of Cardiology* 1991;**67**:1084–9.

59. Bertie J, King A, Reed N, Marshall AJ, Ricketts C. Benefits and weaknesses of a cardiac rehabilitation programme. *Journal of the Royal College of Physicians of London* 1992;**26**:147–51.

60. Kallio V, Cay E (eds). *Rehabilitation after myocardial infarction: the European experience.* Public health in Europe 24. Copenhagen: WHO Regional Office for Europe, 1985.

61. Todd IC, Ballantyne D. The antianginal efficacy of exercise training: a comparison with beta blockade. *British Heart Journal* 1990;**64**:14–9.

62. Coats AJS, Adamopolous S, Meyer TE, Conway J, Sleight P. Effects of physical training in chronic heart failure. *Lancet* 1990;**355**:63–6.

63. Fontana AF, Kerns RD, Rosenberg RL, Colonese KL. Support, stress, and recovery from coronary heart disease: a longitudinal causal model. *Health Psychology* 1989;**8**:175–93.

64. Oldridge NB. Cardiac rehabilitation exercise programme compliance and compliance enhancing strategies. *Sports Medicine* 1988;**6**:42–55.

65. Oldridge NB, Streiner DL. The health belief model: predicting compliance and dropout in cardiac rehabilitation. *Medicine and Science in Sports and Exercise* 1990;**22**:678–83.

66. van Dixhoorn J, Duivenvoorden HJ, Staal HA, Pool J. Physical training and relaxation therapy in cardiac rehabilitation assessed through a composite criterion for training outcome. *American Heart Journal* 1989;**118**:545–52.

67. van Dixhoorn J, Duivenvoorden HJ, Staal HA, *et al.* Cardiac events after myocardial infarction: possible effect of relaxation therapy. *European Heart Journal* 1987;**8**:1210–4.

68. Patel C, Marmot MG, Terry DJ, Carruthers M, *et al.* Trial of relaxation in reducing coronary risk: four year follow-up. *British Medical Journal* 1985;**290**:1103–6.

69. Langosch W. Behavioural interventions in cardiac rehabilitation. In: Steptoe A, Mathews A (eds). *Health care and human behaviour*. London: Academic Press, 1984:301–24.

70. Ornish D, Brown SE, Scherwitz LW, *et al.* Can lifestyle changes reverse coronary heart disease? *Lancet* 1990;**336**:129–33.

71. Sivarajan ES, Newton KM, Almes MJ. Limited effects of outpatient teaching and counselling after myocardial infarction: a controlled study. *Heart and Lung* 1983;**12**:65–73.

72. Barbarowicz P, Nelson M, DeBusk RK, Haskell WL. A comparison of in-hospital education approaches for coronary bypass patients. *Heart and Lung* 1980;**9**:127–33.

73. Martin JE, Dubbert PM. Behavioural management strategies for improving health and fitness. *Journal of Cardiac Rehabilitation* 1984;**4**:200–8.

74. Horlick L, Cameron R, Firor W, Bactzam R, *et al.* The effects of education and group discussion in the post myocardial infarction patient. *Journal of Psychosomatic Research* 1984;**28**:485–92.

75. van Elderen-van Kemenade T, Maes S, van den Broek Y. Effects of a health education programme with telephone follow-up during cardiac rehabilitation. *British Journal of Clinical Psychology* 1994;**33**:367–78.

76. Murray PJ. Rehabilitation information and health beliefs in the post-coronary patient: do we meet their informational needs? *Journal of Advanced Nursing* 1989;**14**:686–93.

77. Freeman LJ, King JC. Sex and the post-infarction patient. *Cardiology in Practice* November 1986:6–8.

78. Taylor CB, Bandura A, Ewart CK. Exercise testing to enhance wives' confidence in their husbands' cardiac capability soon after clinically uncomplicated acute myocardial infarction. *American Journal of Cardiology* 1985;**55**:635–8.

79. Brownell KD, Jeffrey RW. Improving long-term weight loss: pushing the limits of treatment. *Behaviour Therapy* 1987;**18**:353–74.

80. Glasgow RE, Lichtenstein E. Long term effects of behavioural smoking cessation interventions. *Behaviour Therapy* 1987;**18**:297–324.

81. Lovibond SH, Birrell P, Langeluddecke P. Changing coronary heart disease risk-factor status: the effects of three behavioural programmes. *Journal of Behavioral Medicine* 1986;**9**:415–37.

82. Zigmond AS, Snaith RP. The hospital anxiety and depression scale. *Acta Psychiatrica Scandinavica* 1983;**67**:361–70.

83. Goldberg DP. *Detection of psychiatric illness by questionnaire.* London: Oxford University Press, 1972.

84. Mayou R. Prediction of emotional and social outcome after a heart attack. *Journal of Psychosomatic Research* 1984;**28**:17–25.

The social component

Alan Radley
Reader in Health and Social Relations, Department of Social Sciences, Loughborough University

The idea that there should be a social component to cardiac rehabilitation provokes the question 'why?'. What problems are faced by patients in the course of recovery either from a heart attack or from surgical treatment to relieve the symptoms of coronary disease? What kinds of intervention might help them overcome or even avoid these problems?

Before trying to answer these questions, it is essential to note that attention to the social component of cardiac rehabilitation takes us outside medicine. Social matters involve individuals — their bodies and their minds — but are not reducible to these features. The social world is one of disputed judgements and meanings, of shared values and norms. If we seriously want to extend rehabilitation into this sphere, these matters have eventually to be addressed in some detail.

The rationale for considering social aspects is that they impinge upon recovery in ways that make for a better or a worse recovery. This chapter will therefore first consider some of the problems related to cardiac rehabilitation, and then examine the assumptions underlying their investigation to date. This will allow a review of some interventions that concern the social world of the coronary patient, and a discussion of the place of social features in medical treatment for coronary disease.

The problem area approach to rehabilitation

There are three main areas of concern to researchers in the field:

1. Return to work.

2. The relationship of patient with family, especially spouse.

3. Relationships with others, especially friends and confidants (social support).

Return to work

Return to work is discussed fully in Chapter 6, so will be covered only briefly here. The desirability of cardiac patients returning to work is evidenced throughout the literature. Work return has been used as a measure of quality of life; for coronary artery bypass graft surgery, it has stood as one of the initial criteria by which surgical success could be judged. However, it has become evident that whether people return to work depends upon matters other than their physical state after treatment.[1] Readiness to take retirement, the demands of the job, and the availability of disability benefits all affect work return — not to mention the availability of work itself: that is, situational and biographical aspects of life (essentially social features) are important in the decision about return to paid employment. Whether or not patients do return to work, there is evidence (based on male samples) that at least 50% will suffer some financial hardship as a consequence of their illness.[2] Even if work is only temporarily interrupted, the personal financial consequences of heart disease should not be overlooked, as they constrain the possible lines of action that can be taken in the course of recovery.

One distinctly negative outcome is that medical belief in the desirability of return to employment has meant that patients who do not show commitment to do so or who couch their reluctance in terms of concern for their state of health, risk being labelled 'cardiac invalids'.[3] Cardiac rehabilitation is not just about restoring a normal social life to patients; it is also about persuading them to relinquish the sick role (ie to recognise its social undesirability). The best way in which patients can effectively communicate that they have done this is by demonstrating that they can do a full day's work.

Relationships in the family: the role of the spouse/partner

There is now a considerable body of evidence that a heart attack affects the social and emotional life of the patient's family, particularly the spouse.[4-9] This is true both at the time of the attack and in the months (and sometimes years) afterwards. Children are less likely to be affected than spouses in cases where the illness is less apparent, but they too are aware of problems when the patient's illness is more severe.[2] Wives of men who suffer a myocardial infarction (MI) tend to relate the experience to the meaning that their marital relationship has for them.[10] This indicates both the potential for the event to penetrate into every aspect of domestic life, and also how it can affect the social context on which he or she must depend during the time of recovery and rehabilitation.

Heart attacks have a disruptive effect upon the lives of the family, particularly of the spouse, who must continue to run the home against the background of uncertainty about the future. Wives of patients studied demonstrated a need for information to help repair this disruption and to enable them to plan for the future. Immediately after the attack, many wives of patients want information about coronary disease and what it means. At this stage, the patient is likely to be hospitalised, occupies the sick role, and is perceived to be passive in the hands of events and health professionals. During rehabilitation, however, the patient's active role raises questions about the extent and intensity of his commitments. At this later stage, it has been found that wives of heart attack patients want less information about the disease and more about what their husbands should or should not do.[11]

The scope for the spouse to act as helper or as an agent in the course of rehabilitation will be affected in part by the effects of the patient's illness upon the whole family. In this sense, research into the possible role of the spouse (or other family member) in rehabilitation presumes some kind of effect upon the family: that is, what the spouse can do is in part limited by the constraints that have been placed as a result of the family's response to the patient's illness.[12] Among these constraints are the patterns of behaviour habitually adopted by patients and their spouses in the course of solving problems in their relationship. For example, different patterns of exchange between husbands and wives evolve to deal with the difficulties presented by the former's coronary disease.[13] A particular way of coping 'makes sense' in some cases, whereas others will have a different way of managing daily difficulties. This has important consequences for the lines of recovery or rehabilitation envisaged by different couples. For some, a heart attack or the need for bypass surgery is met with opposition and the determination to get back to normal life as quickly as possible; for others, these events present an opportunity to revise not only future plans but also the way in which everyday matters are currently handled.

Research focusing upon male patients and female spouses has shown one pattern of patient-spouse behaviour that presents particular difficulties for rehabilitation (meaning behaviour change). This is when the man is insistent upon retaining an active involvement in everything and the wife is resigned to acceding to his wishes.[13–15] In these relationships, the husbands tend not to report problems and, consistent with this, seek an early return to work.

Their spouses, however, report considerable stress levels, so that the possibility of early resumption of activity by the patient must be set against psychological distress for the spouse.[16] This kind of relationship forms only a minority of those studied, but it has implications for the way in which the patients concerned respond to medical treatment.[17]

This raises questions as to whether efforts at rehabilitation should be aimed at:

- the patient alone,

- the spouse alone (apart from the patient), or

- the patient and spouse together.

There have for some time been programmes aimed at providing the spouse and other carers with a forum in which they can discuss their particular problems.[3,18] It has also been recognised that spouses can offer help as well as take it.[19]

It has been argued that spouse support is integral to compliance by the patient to regimens and life adjustments after infarction.[20] However, it should not be assumed that all patient-spouse behaviour is, of necessity, supportive or constructive. Research in the context of pain has found that overinvolvement by or too much support from the spouse can hinder rehabilitation.[21] Also, needs change as rehabilitation progresses, so a patient-spouse agreement that is constructive in the early stages of recovery can become unhelpful when there is a recovery of normal life.[22]

Particularly in those cases in which male cardiac patients are insistently active and their spouse/partner repeatedly tries (but fails) to modify their levels of activity, a cycle of behaviour is maintained that eludes intervention.[13] Behaviour patterns in the home are resistant to change from outside — one reason, perhaps, why attempts to modify individual risk behaviour, through either directive advice[23] or discussion groups,[24] have so far met with limited success.

An alternative technique that has been tried with these ('difficult') men by Hoebel[25] is to modify the patient-spouse behaviour pattern of exchange rather than the actions of the patient as an individual. Their wives were recruited to a programme of action in which they did not try to dissuade, cajole or otherwise direct their husbands towards medically approved goals. Instead, they were explicitly pessimistic about their husbands' efforts at risk-reducing behaviour. Once deprived of their wives' attempts to control them, these patients undertook for themselves the behaviours that they had so long been struggling to avoid.

This specific programme might be suitable only for certain kinds of patient-spouse relationship, but it indicates that any kind of rehabilitation must continue in the context of domestic life. This has a variety of forms, so it is unlikely that any one intervention will always be successful. Hoebel's work also suggests that spouses should not be involved only as an addition to the focus on the patient, but that the spouse-patient *relationship* might well be the appropriate focus for some of the rehabilitative work that health professionals wish to undertake.

Relationships with friends and confidants

Different people will be of help to patients and carers at different points in the patient's recovery. Social support is important, but it is necessary to remember that the definition of an 'able-bodied' person in society is someone who can give, as well as receive, help. A randomised controlled trial of cardiac rehabilitation patients found that moderating social support (ie maintaining the patient's independence within the family) contributed to work resumption.[26] The idea that other people beyond the immediate family also have a role in the rehabilitation of the cardiac patient is well documented.[2,27–29] One longitudinal study[30] showed that such support ameliorated the accompanying experience of stress and distress, and had opposite effects on cardiac symptoms to those variables. In addition, it was noted that support was more influential in the first six months following hospitalisation for a heart attack — under-lining the point that 'need varies over time', and that the movement towards good health is directed away from being perceived by others as requiring assistance. The process of normalising one's heart attack[7,31] — of making it 'sensible' — goes on after discharge from hospital, when friends and colleagues play an important role in re-establishing the patient as a 'normal' healthy person.

This change in health status is important to achieve, given the widespread belief among the general public that, following a heart attack, the person concerned should considerably limit his or her activity.[3] In the light of this notion, it is not surprising to learn that patients see their social relationships as providing both hindrances and aids towards achieving a steady recovery.[29]

Features of relationships that *hinder* the motivation of patients to engage in desirable behaviour include:

- conflict between their own and others' values; and

- being monitored by others in the family.[29]

The *helpful* features include:

- emotional support, which can be provided by health professionals, other patients and friends — by being available and showing that they care and will listen, other people have a key role in encouraging patients, particularly in the early stages of recovery;

- appraisal support, through which others give consistent feed-back and encouragement regarding goals and performance; and

- problem-solving, involving sharing knowledge so that patients can be well informed and helped to explore alternative lines of action.

These three different kinds of enabling support are available to varying degrees from professionals,[27,32] other patients[15,33,34] and associates. In particular, emotional support is seen by patients to relate to secure and coherent relationships with their spouse-partner.[35] The forms of support available will depend upon the social network of the patient concerned.[28] It has been shown that different ways of adjusting to the patient's cardiac illness are tried out by the patient and spouse together,[15] relating to the social networks of the individual couples. Patients and spouses who rely mainly upon family cope differently together to couples who draw upon a network of friends and associates. Although no single pattern of support is essentially better than another, it seems that severe lack of support is related to poorer outcome, both psychological[15,29] and in terms of survival in later years.[36]

Examination of assumptions behind the problem-centred approach

The research flowing from the problem-centred approach suggests lines of intervention, but it is important to recognise its limitations. Three, in particular, will be mentioned, each arising from an unwarranted tendency to generalise from specific patient groups.

Gender differences

Gender differences have largely been overlooked.[37] Most studies have been of male patients, so 'spouses' invariably means 'wives'. Women respond differently to coronary disease:

- They are more likely to withdraw from the labour market;[38]

this cannot be explained in terms of disease severity, but appears to be related to the kinds of social expectations with which they are faced.

■ They are less likely to attend rehabilitation programmes, for reasons not yet fully clear.[39] One reason is the 'sex role' — again relating to the social expectations that attach to women and to what they are expected to do and not do.

■ There is evidence that women cardiac patients approach the period following their heart attack in a different way to men.[40]

There is, however, also evidence that older women and older men do not differ in emotional well-being and psychosocial functioning, as related to the self-management of their cardiac illness.[41] Nevertheless, women have particular expectations, and their spouses/partners have expectations of them, which are not reducible to a set of needs derived from the study of men alone. There is very little information about the husband/partner as carer.

The social significance of ageing

Studies of cardiac rehabilitation have not always taken due account of the social significance of ageing. It has been shown among college students[42] that age stereotypes are more pronounced than gender stereotypes, and that the two often work together.[43] The implication is that rehabilitation programmes should at least examine the assumptions made about the aspirations, experience and abilities of the patients. In particular, it was shown in a sample of older cardiac patients that cardiac symptoms decreased in the men over the first year post-MI, while those of the women increased.[44] The authors of this report suggested that older women have social and medical disadvantages that deserve special attention from professionals devising coronary rehabilitation programmes.

Heterogeneity of patients

The criticism has been made that analysis of the effects of cardiac rehabilitation is hampered by the heterogeneity of the patients.[45] This appears as a criticism when seen from the perspective of biomedical research using natural science methodology but, if the points about gender and age are taken into account, the social setting of the patient becomes more, not less, important — something to inquire into, not try to exclude as an error variable. Hospital programmes have approached rehabilitation from a broadly biomedical perspective, which is inappropriate to the domestic and wider social setting. The kinds of studies needed to plan programmes that extend into the community are still rare in the literature.[46,47] Although heterogeneity appears as a methodological problem for experimental research, it is basic to studies of the social component of rehabilitation.

The social component reassessed

The social component of cardiac rehabilitation, as reflected in many studies, refers to patients' work status, leisure activities and contacts with other people. This view implies that what is 'social' is somehow beyond the individual, outside the psychological and the physical: having got the patient to exercise, and then sorted out his or her anxieties, that patient can then be returned to normal life in the community.

The assumption that rehabilitation builds up from the physical, through exercise programmes, via the psychological to the social is a flawed vision. For example, the assumption that the psychological benefits of rehabilitation classes are mediated by changes in physical fitness has been questioned.[48] The values, hopes and fears that patients bring to any rehabilitation class (and outside) have their roots in the kinds of lives patients lead with others. The social component is not a shell surrounding the physical and the psychological; it penetrates these spheres, so that whether and how people exercise and what they fear about their illness relate to the things in their everyday lives that matter to them. Thus, the social component to cardiac rehabilitation is always present, even when investigators have not built it into their research designs.

A second assumption about the social component must be questioned. From the biomedical point of view, the patient is a passive recipient of treatment and rehabilitation. Health professionals have the knowledge that allows them to make interventions in that patient's life. However, what appears to the medical researcher as a social component, a variable that can be acted upon, is an integral part of the biography of the patient. Far from being passive objects, patients have their own expectations about their illness and what can be done about it. These have been shown to be *better* predictors of return to work and general functioning in the six months after hospitalisation than the medical models of their physician:[49] that is, patients are busy making sense of their life and their illness in ways that cannot be ignored if we wish to help them make a full recovery. The literature on 'patient compliance' is littered with discarded studies that assumed people can be treated as passive receivers of guidance from experts (see Ref 50).

What can be done about 'social' rehabilitation?

Three summary points may be made from this overview of the social component of cardiac rehabilitation:

1. Aspects of the social context are known, some relating to a better and others to a worse prognosis after a heart attack. Having a caring and supportive family, good friends and a job to which the patient wants to return are all conducive to a positive recovery. The problem is that these aspects are not amenable to medical intervention. Also, many people in Britain today live on their own, do not have a job (let alone a rewarding one) and perhaps only a few friends. Generalised findings about these social variables are of little help in a world of varied social situations.

   Against this background, it is unwise — if not ethically dubious — for health professionals to promulgate certain lifestyles as desirable and others as undesirable when they cannot give the people concerned the wherewithal to change their situation.

2. One line of action sometimes recommended is to target for special attention patients who are at-risk in terms of their demographic status. For example, socially isolated patients might be selected for counselling about their progress when they leave hospital. This targeting of patients by means of social indicators, however, carries the risk of projecting on to certain groups the assumptions built into the models used by health researchers. For example, what might begin as a laudable attempt to 'get patients back to work' ends up focusing upon individuals labelled as 'malingerers' or 'cardiac invalids'. Individuals who do not fit into the aims of a social rehabilitation programme can too easily become stigmatised by the very groups who wish to help them. Instead, we have to understand how patients come to see certain lines of action as 'normal' or 'undesirable' in the light of (or in spite of) the information they are given.

3. From what has been said above, clearly the social component of cardiac rehabilitation does not start when the patient leaves hospital. From the time of admission onwards, work, home and friends all fill in the patient's concerns about what has

happened and what will happen.[31] The challenge for health workers is to discover how these matters affect the course of patients' progress through the system. How patients make sense of their own social situations will impinge upon standardised interventions such as exercise programmes. Health workers can then help patients (and their spouses/partners) to articulate their concerns, and to establish how they can best use medical information and advice.

While this is not difficult to do, for example, by means of discussion groups involving spouses/partners, its efficacy is more difficult to prove. The disrupted judgements and shared values of the social world are more open-ended than the fixed aims of physical and psychological rehabilitation would allow. Within a research tradition that gives strict approval only to randomised control designs, the patient's view (not to mention that of the group) appears subjective and impossible to investigate. If this means that these matters are not studied, the 'social component' in cardiac rehabilitation will remain a feature which health professionals aspire to involve in their work, but the inclusion of which they can never fully justify.

References

1. Oberman A, Wayne JB, Kouchoukos NT, Charles ED, *et al.* Employment status after coronary bypass surgery. *Circulation* 1982;**65**(Suppl 3):115–9.

2. Croog SH, Levine S. *Life after a heart attack: social and psychological factors eight years later.* New York: Human Sciences Press, 1982.

3. Monteiro LA. *Cardiac patient rehabilitation: social aspects of recovery.* New York: Springer, 1979.

4. Mayou R, Foster A, Williamson B. The psychological and social effects of myocardial infarction on wives. *British Medical Journal* 1978;**1**:699–701.

5. McGee HM, Graham T, Newton H, Horgan JH. The involvement of the spouse in cardiac rehabilitation. *Irish Journal of Psychology* 1994;**15**:203–18.

6. Skelton M, Dominion J. Psychological stress in wives of patients with myocardial infarction. *British Medical Journal* 1973;**2**:101–3.

7. Speedling EJ. *Heart attack: the family response at home and in the hospital.* New York, London: Tavistock, 1982.

8. Thompson DR, Cordle CJ. Support of wives of myocardial infarction patients. *Journal of Advanced Nursing* 1988;**13**:223–8.

9. Thompson DR, Meddis R. Wives' responses to counselling early after myocardial infarction. *Journal of Psychosomatic Research* 1990;**34**:249–58.

10. Michela JL. Interpersonal and individual impacts of a husband's heart attack. In: Baum A, Singer J (eds). *Handbook of psychology and health, vol 5: Stress and coping.* Hillsdale, NJ: Lawrence Erlbaum Associates, 1987:255–300.

11. Doherty ES, Power PW. Identifying the needs of coronary patient wife-caregivers: implications for social workers. *Health and Social Work* 1990;**15**:291–9.

12. Bermann E. Regrouping for survival: approaching dread and three phases of family interaction. *Journal of Comparative and Family Studies* 1973;**4**:63–87.

13. Radley A, Green R. Bearing illness: a study of couples where the husband awaits coronary graft surgery. *Social Science and Medicine* 1986;**23**:577–85.

14. Helgeson VS. Implications of agency and communion for patient and spouse adjustment to a first coronary event. *Journal of Personality and Social Psychology* 1993;**64**:807–16.

15. Radley A. *Prospects of heart surgery: psychological adjustment to coronary bypass grafting*. New York: Springer-Verlag, 1988.

16. Radley A, Green R, Radley M. Impending surgery: the expectations of male coronary patients and their wives. *International Rehabilitation Medicine* 1987;**8**:154–61.

17. Bruce EH, Bruce RA, Hossack KF, Kusumi F. Psychosocial coping strategies and cardiac capacity before and after coronary bypass surgery. *International Journal of Psychiatry in Medicine* 1983;**13**:69–84.

18. Gillis CL. Reducing family stress during and after coronary artery bypass surgery. *Nursing Clinics of North America* 1984;**19**:103–12.

19. Acker JE, McMorran PR, Friedlob JW, Wade CC. Assessing psychological problems from a cardiologist's point of view. *Advances in Cardiology* 1982;**31**: 218–22.

20. Miller PJ, Wikoff R. Spouses' psychological problems, resources, and marital functioning post myocardial infarction. *Progress in Cardiovascular Nursing* 1989;**4**:71–6.

21. Block AR, Boyer SL. The spouse's adjustment to chronic pain: cognitive and emotional factors. *Social Science and Medicine* 1984;**19**:1313–7.

22. Bar-On D, Dreman S. When spouses disagree: a predictor of cardiac rehabilitation. *Family Systems Medicine* 1987;**5**:228–37.

23. Family Heart Study Group. Randomised controlled trial evaluating cardiovascular screening and intervention in general practice, principal results of British family heart study. *British Medical Journal* 1994;**308**:313–20.

24. Horlick L, Cameron R, Firor W, *et al.* The effects of education and group discussion in the post myocardial infarction patient. *Journal of Psychosomatic Research* 1984;**28**:485–92.

25. Hoebel FC. Coronary artery disease and family interaction: a study of risk factor modification. In: Watzlawick P, Weakland JH (eds). *The interactional view: studies at the Mental Research Institute, Paulo Alto, 1965–74*. New York: Norton, 1977.

26. Burgess AW, Lerner DJ, D'Agostino RB, Vokonas PS, *et al.* A randomised control trial of cardiac rehabilitation. *Social Science and Medicine* 1987;**24**:359–70.

27. Bramwell L. Social support in cardiac rehabilitation. *Canadian Journal of Cardiovascular Nursing* 1990;**1**:7–13.

28. Finlayson A. Social networks as coping resources. *Social Science and Medicine* 1976;**10**:97–103.

29. Fleury J. An exploration of the role of social networks in cardiovascular risk reduction. *Heart and Lung* 1993;**22**:134–44.

30. Fontana AF, Kerns RD, Rosenberg RL, Colonese KL. Support, stress and recovery from coronary heart disease: a longitudinal model. *Health Psychology* 1989;**8**:175–93.

31. Cowie B. The cardiac patient's perception of his heart attack. *Social Science and Medicine* 1976;**10**:87–96.

32. Winefield HR, Katsikis M. Medical professional support and cardiac rehabilitation of males and females. *Journal of Psychosomatic Research* 1987;**31**:567–73.

33. Meagher DM, Gregor F, Stewart M. Dyadic social-support for cardiac surgery patients — a Canadian approach. *Social Science and Medicine* 1987;**25**:833–7.

34. Simpson R. Relationships between self-help organizations and professional health care providers. *Health and Social Care in the Community* 1996;**4**:359–70.

35. Waltz M. Marital context and post-infarction quality of life: is it social support or something more? *Social Science and Medicine* 1986;**22**:791–805.

36. Ruberman E, Weinblatt E, Goldberg JD, Chaudary BS. Psychosocial influences on mortality after myocardial infarction. *New England Journal of Medicine* 1984;**311**:552–9.

37. Khaw KT. Where are the women in studies of coronary heart disease? *British Medical Journal* 1993;**306**:1145–6.

38. Chirikos TN, Nickel JL. Work disability from coronary heart disease in women. *Women and Health* 1984;**9**:55–74.

39. McGee HM, Horgan JH. Cardiac rehabilitation programmes: are women less likely to attend? *British Medical Journal* 1992;**305**:283–4.

40. Boogaard MAK. Rehabilitation of the female patient after myocardial infarction. *Symposium on Current Topics in Cardiac Nursing* 1984;**19**:433–9.

41. Sharpe PA, Clark NM, Janz NK. Differences in the impact and management of heart disease between older women and men. *Women and Health* 1991;**17**:25–43.

42. Kite ME, Deaux K, Miele M. Stereotypes of young and old: does age outweigh gender? *Psychology and Aging* 1991;**6**:19–27.

43. Hockey J, James A. *Growing up and growing old: ageing and dependency in the life course.* London: Sage, 1993.

44. Young RF, Kahana E. Gender, recovery from late life heart attack, and medical care. *Women and Health* 1993;**20**:11–31.

45. Lipkin DP (editorial). Is cardiac rehabilitation necessary? *British Heart Journal* 1991;**65**:237–8.

46. Finlayson A, McEwen J. *Coronary heart disease and patterns of living.* New York: Prodist, 1977.

47. Jacobson MM, Eichhorn RL. How families cope with heart disease: a study of problems and resources. *Journal of Marriage and the Family* 1964;**26**: 166–73.

48. Rovario S, Holmes DS, Holmsten RD. Influence of a cardiac rehabilitation program on the cardiovascular, psychological and social functioning of cardiac patients. *Journal of Behavioral Medicine* 1984;**7**:61–81.

49. Bar-On D. Professional models vs patient models in rehabilitation after heart attack. *Human Relations* 1986;**39**:917–32.

50. Stimson G. Obeying doctor's orders: a view from the other side. *Social Science and Medicine* 1974;**8**:97–104.

5 The exercise component

Adrianne Hardman

Reader in Human Exercise Metabolism, Department of Physical Education, Sports Science and Recreation Management, Loughborough University

Exercise training contributes to the rehabilitation of patients with coronary heart disease (CHD) by counteracting the deleterious effects of bed-rest, and by improving both exercise tolerance and the responses to submaximal exertion, in particular by reducing myocardial oxygen demands. Additional gains which may influence the likelihood of further clinical episodes are favourable alterations in several risk factors and, when combined with a lipid-lowering diet, possibly a reduction in the progression of the underlying coronary atherosclerosis.

Over the last decade the pathophysiological severity of acute illness has been changed by earlier and more intensive interventions during the acute phase of the disease, particularly thrombolysis, with or without subsequent angioplasty or coronary artery bypass graft (CABG) surgery. There is less myocardial damage and residual ischaemia, and therefore less myocardial dysfunction, so physical exercise rehabilitation can be initiated earlier.

This chapter will describe the physiological and metabolic adaptations which result in improved functional capacity and endurance (stamina), and consider the efficacy, safety and applicability of different approaches to exercise training.

Physiological and metabolic adaptations to endurance (aerobic) training

Marked cardiovascular, metabolic, thermoregulatory and hormonal adjustments occur during a bout of exercise. It is important to realise that these are not related to the *absolute* intensity of the exercise, measured by its oxygen demand and proportional to work rate or speed of walking or running, for example, but to the intensity *relative to individual functional capacity*. Functional capacity is best measured by the maximal oxygen uptake ($\dot{v}O_2$max) (or peak performance). For weight-bearing exercise, which covers most daily life activities, this is most usefully expressed per kg of body mass.

Exercise sufficient to stimulate a 'training effect' will, if performed regularly and frequently, result in a higher $\dot{V}O_2$max. It also stimulates adaptive changes in the trained skeletal muscles, delaying the onset of fatigue and improving endurance (ie the capability to sustain for a reasonable period without fatigue exercise which constitutes a high proportion of personal $\dot{V}O_2$max). Although peak performance is important because it provides a reserve for unexpected demands, improved endurance is the more important physiological goal for most patients.

CHD patients typically show a substantial improvement in $\dot{V}O_2$max during rehabilitation, the biggest improvements tending to be in those patients with the lowest initial values: 11–56% in patients recovering from acute myocardial infarction (MI), and usually more (14–66%) in CABG patients after 3–6 months of exercise training.[1] Improvements are frequently of a greater magnitude than those seen in apparently healthy individuals because of the contribution of the natural process of recovery from infarction or surgery and the effect of resumption of routine physical activities.

In healthy, normally active individuals, central (cardiovascular) and peripheral (metabolic) adaptations both contribute to training-induced increases in $\dot{V}O_2$max.[2] In cardiac patients, these increases are predominantly a result of adaptations in the trained skeletal muscle, resulting in increased oxygen extraction and utilisation — and, therefore, in an increased arteriovenous difference.[3] The oxidative capacity of trained skeletal muscle is enhanced because of greater activity of mitochondrial enzymes[4] and, in the longer term, possible improvements in the microcirculation.[5] Collectively, these improvements are manifest in less dependence on glycolysis during submaximal exercise and, in turn, in a reduced blood lactate response. Increases in muscle oxidative capacity occur rapidly with the onset of training, with associated rapid improvements in endurance; conversely, these adaptations are rapidly lost when training ceases.

Central myocardial adaptations have been demonstrated in patients after MI,[6] but these investigators studied prolonged (≥ 1 year) and intense (ca 85% $\dot{V}O_2$max) training. Improvements in left ventricular contractile function were evident from increased ejection fraction, stroke volume and rate pressure product during maximal exercise.

When $\dot{V}O_2$max is enhanced by training, a given submaximal exercise represents a smaller proportion of functional capacity, so endurance is improved and there is less fatigue. Improvements in endurance are disproportionately greater than parallel increases in

$\dot{V}O_2$max, and are manifestly rewarding for the patient. Many responses to standardised submaximal exercise are altered by training. Examples are:

- the classic bradycardia, which is readily evident and, together with the reduction in systolic blood pressure, means a reduction in myocardial work and therefore in oxygen demand;

- changes in exercise-induced redistribution of cardiac output; and

- a smaller rise in deep body temperature.

All such changes probably contribute to a reduction in the individual's perception of the severity of a given submaximal exercise.

The lower heart rate during exercise is attributed to a reduced sympathetic response (evident in lower plasma noradrenaline concentrations) and possibly increased vagal tone. These adaptations are particularly important for patients with exertional ischaemia because they raise the level of exercise which will precipitate symptoms to a similar extent as that achieved by beta-blockade.[7] A recent study in men under the age of 60 with stable angina, but no previous MI, found that the number and duration of painful episodes of ischaemia were reduced after one year following a daily callisthenic exercise programme.[8] Reported improvements in symptom-limited $\dot{V}O_2$max in patients with angina pectoris range from 32–56%.[1]

Secondary prevention of coronary heart disease events

Improved survival has been an important outcome measure for assessing the benefit of rehabilitation. An overview[9] of 22 randomised trials of cardiac rehabilitation which included structured exercise indicated a moderate reduction of about 20% in total and cardiovascular-related mortality, with a particularly large reduction (odds ratio, 0.63; 95% confidence interval, 0.41–0.97) for sudden death. A similar meta-analysis of 10 trials[10] found a 25% reduction in cardiovascular mortality associated with cardiac rehabilitation. These reductions are of a similar order to those achieved by prophylactic beta-blockade.

The evidence is, however, inconclusive as to whether exercise *independently* affects the likelihood of reinfarction: none of the relatively small number of randomised 'exercise-only' trials had the statistical power to demonstrate a possible protective effect of exercise. Regular physical activity has repeatedly been shown to play an independent role in reducing the risk of experiencing a *first* clinical episode of CHD in asymptomatic middle-aged men,[11] even among those at high risk.[12]

Mechanisms

Possible protective mechanisms include effects on both the chronic and the acute phases of the disease. In patients with stable angina pectoris, the progression of CHD, as assessed by changes in the diameter of coronary lesions visualised angiographically, was slower in those undertaking exercise training combined with a low-fat, lipid-lowering diet than in comparable controls.[13,14] Enhanced dilatation of coronary arteries is a more speculative suggestion. This has been reported in male marathon runners,[15] but it is not known whether moderate exercise would produce this in patients with coronary atherosclerosis. A recent observation that exercise-induced platelet activation occurs in sedentary people, but not in physically active people,[16] provides a plausible explanation for the protective effect of regular exercise on acute thromboembolytic events.

Outcome measures

As Wenger pointed out,[17] in the future there will probably be less emphasis on improved survival and reduced rates of reinfarction as outcome variables for rehabilitative care, at least for low-risk patients. Exercise may not offer much likelihood of short-term survival or reinfarction benefit above that conferred by current therapeutic interventions such as thrombolysis, improved pharmacotherapy and myocardial revascularisation procedures. The emphasis will increasingly be on quality of life measures. Thus, improvements in functional capacity and endurance, and the increased self-confidence which accrue, are likely to be the benefits on which a rationale for exercise in rehabilitation is predicated.

Influence on risk factors

Endurance training has well documented effects on risk factors for CHD, but these effects have been most clearly demonstrated in healthy volunteers. One reason for this is the need for a 'lifestyle' approach to rehabilitation, in which advice on stopping smoking and dietary change is inevitably given in parallel with exercise prescription. This makes it difficult to isolate the contribution of exercise to other changes in behaviour.

Lipoproteins

Based on studies of healthy people, endurance training (but not strength training) results in favourable changes in lipoprotein metabolism, in particular, increases in serum high-density lipo-protein (HDL) cholesterol and decreases in triacylglycerol.[18–20] The 'dosage' of exercise needed to be effective to increase HDL cholesterol is uncertain, although it has been proposed that a minimum exercise energy expenditure of 1,000–1,200 kcal per week over at least six months is necessary.[18,20] It may well be less for recently bed-rested patients. Changes in the chemical composition of low-density lipoprotein may also occur — making this lipoprotein species more cholesterol-rich and protein-poor.[21]

If a primary therapeutic goal is to decrease serum total choles-terol, exercise may not be the therapy of choice. A lower total chol-esterol concentration may, however, be an *indirect* benefit from exer-cise: as physical activity levels increase, there is a tendency for the proportion of energy consumed as carbohydrate to increase, with a complementary decrease in energy obtained from fat and a fall in total cholesterol concentration. For patients on beta-blockade, exercise may be helpful in reducing the deterioration in the lipid profile known to occur with this therapy.[22]

Insulin/glucose dynamics

It has been recognised recently that the changes in lipoprotein metabolism may be linked to decreased insulin resistance.[23] This brings greater inhibition of non-esterified fatty acid release from adipose tissue during the postprandial period and an enhanced uptake of triacylglycerol-rich lipoproteins. Both effects could be invoked to explain the low levels of postprandial lipaemia demonstrated in athletes;[24] the latter effect will also result in a greater transfer of surface material to HDL, possibly enhancing 'reverse cholesterol transport'.

Enhanced insulin sensitivity is evident with endurance training, although it is uncertain whether this is independent of the effects of the last bout of exercise.[25,26] Skeletal muscle is the body's largest insulin-sensitive tissue, so increases in insulin sensitivity will be quantitatively important. The decreases in body weight and fatness associated with both endurance and strength training[27] are probably also important, as are the increases in muscle mass *per se*.

Blood pressure

Resting blood pressure is lowered by endurance training and circuit training (exercises designed to increase both strength and endurance) in hypertensive and normotensive people, the average reduction in the better-designed studies being 6–7 mmHg for both systolic and diastolic pressures.[28] Low to moderate intensity exercise may well be more effective than intense exercise in this regard.[29] Strength training may not reduce blood pressure, at least in older people.[30]

Effects of each exercise bout

Awareness has recently increased of the importance of the effects of *each* bout of exercise for cardiovascular risk. Even light exercise increases the metabolic rate profoundly; for example, walking at 3 mph increases energy expenditure above the resting level more than threefold to about 4.5 kcal per min. Metabolism remains high for some time after exercise, the magnitude of the increase depending on its intensity and duration. Insulin sensitivity is enhanced for at least some hours following a bout of exercise,[31] probably reflecting changes in the exercised skeletal muscle. This has sometimes been regarded as a means of enhancing muscle glucose uptake to replenish glycogen stores depleted by intense exercise, but a recent report of lower insulin concentrations for several hours following walking[32] — light exercise and therefore not glycogen depleting — suggests that this may not be the only explanation.

Serum triacylglycerol concentration decreases during recovery from exercise.[33] This results from changes in the dynamic exchange of triacylglycerol and cholesterol between lipoproteins, arising from the exercise-stimulated increased activity of lipoprotein lipase in exercised skeletal muscle. This enzyme hydrolyses triacylglycerol in chylomicrons and very low density lipoproteins at the capillary endothelium in muscle and adipose tissue. When the activity of lipoprotein lipase is enhanced, triacylglycerol removal rates increase, with an increase in the rate of HDL synthesis, and triacylglycerol-rich lipoproteins persist for a shorter time in the circulation. These effects can be demonstrated clearly in the post-prandial state when even light exercise markedly attenuates the lipaemic response to dietary fat.[34]

Thus, the insulinaemic and lipaemic responses to a meal are attenuated for some hours after each bout of moderate exercise, so patients can take exercise before a meal and reduce the increase in the cardiovascular risks associated with the postprandial period. There may be a secondary benefit from the reduced lipaemia if the haemostatic changes associated with the postprandial state are attenuated.

The exercise programme

Some comments about the nature of the recommended exercise regimen may be made on the basis of the above consideration of the 'chronic' and 'acute' responses to exercise. Endurance (aerobic) exercise training should be the major component. Large increases in energy expenditure can be achieved and sustained for some time without fatigue once the individual becomes accustomed to an increased level of exercise, and it demands a high cardiac output for a prolonged period.

The body's large muscle groups should be employed in a dynamic way. Local vasodilatation causes a fall in peripheral resistance; this opposes the rise in blood pressure otherwise associated with increased cardiac output, thus increasing safety. Benefits, short- and long-term, associated with peripheral metabolic changes localised to the trained muscles, are also maximised when the muscle mass employed is large.

It is advisable to include various modes of exercise (eg cycling, rowing, walking), which will both minimise the problems of injury and maximise peripheral benefits, as well as maintain variety and therefore patient motivation.

Frequency of exercise

Some of the metabolic effects of exercise appear to be relatively short-lived, so cardiac patients should exercise frequently, even daily, for optimal benefit. A minimum of 3–4 bouts per week is needed to sustain more favourable glucose/insulin dynamics — probably also for the improved lipaemic response to dietary fat. This exercise frequency should be attainable after six months of participation. There are implications here for hospital-based rehabilitation, but it is clearly important that in the longer term patients must choose exercise that they are likely to engage in *frequently* and *continue* over their lifetime.

Intensity of exercise

The issue of exercise intensity is critical for risk-benefit assessment because vigorous exercise carries a high risk of precipitating MI.[35,36] Benefit, in terms of a substantially lower incidence of first coronary events in asymptomatic men, is associated with *moderate* activity like walking and cycling.[12,37,38] It is plausible to suggest that this may also be true for patients. New data show that a satisfactory training effect can result from exercise regimens of moderate intensity, compensated by longer duration and greater frequency,[17] an approach that:

- is associated with better adherence;

- is characterised by greater safety, because patients exercise further from their ischaemic threshold;

- can be undertaken with less professional supervision, and is therefore less costly; and

- fosters the important progressive transition to independence in exercising.

It is the intensity of the exercise *relative to* $\dot{v}O_2$max that dictates the degree of 'physiological stress' experienced. Caution and discretion should therefore be exerted in the prescription of exercise intensity until some assessment of functional capacity can be made, where possible through a graded exercise test. The prescription should be based on the patient's clinical status and related to the predetermined functional capacity, which can range from 50–85%. High-intensity exercise will produce optimal levels of fitness, but many benefits will be evident from less than optimal levels, and there may be both clinical and motivational reasons for not prescribing exercise at the top end of the range.

Three different methods of prescribing and monitoring exercise intensity have been described comprehensively by the American College of Sports Medicine[39] from:

- heart rate,

- ratings of perceived exertion, and

- knowledge of the estimated 'metabolic cost' of activities (multiples of resting metabolic rate (METs) (1 MET = oxygen consumed by awake individual at rest = 3.5 ml/kg/min).

All three methods should be regarded as guidelines only and be modified according to the individual response.

Duration of exercise

The duration of exercise may vary, but it is typically 20–30 min. This period has been regarded as the minimum time, regularly under-taken, needed to improve or maintain functional capacity. Recent evidence, however, has suggested that this goal may be achieved as effectively with more shorter (15 min) bouts as with fewer longer bouts. This approach may be appropriate for home-based prescription. As with other exercise variables, the duration of each session needs to be increased very gradually, from initial sessions as short as 5 min.

Need for strength training?

Provided that a range of different muscle groups are trained, endurance exercise will confer sufficiently good levels of strength for the activities of daily living for many patients. For those whose occu-pational work is manual, some specific training to improve strength may be indicated. In the past, isometric exercise (which maximises strength gains) was avoided because of the marked increases in left ventricular pressure and arrhythmias which were provoked. Recent studies, however, have demonstrated that strength can be increased safely through isometric and resistive exercise, provided that the intensity of the exercise is kept low.[40] All patients should undergo a background of endurance training — ideally, a minimum of four months[41] — before attempting to improve strength: if this is desired, a low-resistance, high-repetition schedule should be followed to stimulate a degree of muscle hypertrophy, whilst keeping the exercise-induced rise in blood pressure to a minimum. Upper body strength is likely to be important to prepare for return to manual occupational work, but needs particular care.

Resistive weight lifting at up to 100% of maximal contraction has recently been shown to provoke a more favourable myocardial oxygen supply-to-demand balance (assessed as the ratio of diastolic pressure-time index to rate-pressure product) than that induced by maximal treadmill exercise, showing that this exercise may not always be contraindicated.[41] This report, however, was in selected, clinically stable, aerobically trained patients with adequate ventricular function, and other patients may respond differently. Most patients will have no need to attempt this level of resistive training.

Phases of exercise rehabilitation

Four phases are generally recognised:

- *Phase I:* the hospital in-patient period

- *Phase II:* the convalescent stage following discharge

- *Phase III:* supervised rehabilitation

- *Phase IV:* unsupervised maintenance programme with outpatient review.

Different proposals have been made for the specific components of these phases,[1,42] but common elements are that there should be early mobilisation in Phase I, with risk assessment or stratification either in Phase I or within a few weeks of leaving hospital. The latter will depend on assessment of the extent of myocardial damage, left ventricular function, and the presence or absence of residual myocardial ischaemia and ventricular arrhythmias. Detailed recommendations for exercise prescription at each stage are reported elsewhere.[39,43]

Low-risk patients

One-third to one-half of those who have experienced MI are low-risk patients, as are about three-quarters of those who have undergone CABG.[1] These patients probably do not need electrocardiographic (ECG)-monitored exercise and can exercise independently after basic instruction. There is no consensus about whether adherence is better or worse with supervised or unsupervised exercise. The resulting improvement in functional capacity is comparable, although supervised programmes may achieve this more rapidly because they tend to enjoy higher training intensities. Social factors, as well as the patient's prior experience of exercise, appear to be important in determining adherence. Subsets of patients, for example, cigarette smokers and overweight individuals, are less likely to adhere to an exercise programme.

High-risk patients

High-risk patients with, for example, exercised-induced hypo-tension, low left ventricular ejection fraction (<35%) or functional capacity below 6 METs, require more extensive monitoring. In practice, because of the number of patients below the 6 MET threshold, these criteria may have to be modified. Those who cannot monitor their own heart rate or who habitually exceed their recommended heart rate range may also need to be regarded as high risk for this purpose.[17]

Supervised or unsupervised programmes?

In ideal circumstances, a well-designed home exercise programme may result in as much exercise being performed as in clinically-based programmes, but the social support of group programmes may be important to many participants.

During the first months following MI or surgery the majority of patients will require hospital-based, supervised exercise because of the need for health care personnel to be present for exercise guidance, monitoring of heart rate, blood pressure, ECG, compliance with the exercise prescription, and emergency care. After this period it will be important to cater for the needs and preferences of individual patients, some of whom will fare better with continued group support, whilst others will achieve more exercise through a flexible, home-based prescription. Safety has to be the overriding concern, but unrealistic estimates of the hazards of moderate exercise should not be invoked, thus denying patients the many benefits which may accrue.

Longer-term supervised programmes may be particularly useful for higher-risk patients, those who perform heavy occupational work and those who need reinforcement to make the behavioural changes needed for risk factor modification.[1] The need for ECG telemetry during supervised programmes has been examined. A large-scale survey[44] found no significant differences in the rates of cardiac arrest, recurrent MI or fatality between programmes with different extents of ECG monitoring. These were defined as continuous, intermittent or graduated (ie continuous for up to three sessions, progressing to intermittent). Recent American College of Cardiology guidelines therefore call for monitoring only in moderate- or high-risk patients fulfilling defined criteria — mainly clinical, but also including an inability to self-monitor exercise heart rate.[45]

Safety

The most comprehensive study of the incidence of cardiovascular complications during rehabilitation is based on data obtained from 167 randomly selected programmes throughout the US involving over 51,000 patients:[44] 21 cardiac arrests (3 fatal) and eight non-fatal MIs were reported. The rate of complications was one cardiac arrest per 111,996 hours of prescribed, supervised exercise, one acute MI per 293,900 hours, and one fatality per 783,976 hours. This relatively high level of safety cannot be taken for granted and undoubtedly reflects careful patient evaluation, treatment and exercise prescription, with appropriate ECG monitoring, well-trained personnel, and rapid, effective handling of emergencies. Concerns other than patient safety may influence decisions about the level of monitoring; for example, the need to demonstrate that safeguards were in place, in the event of an exercise-triggered complication or death.

The safety of home-based rehabilitation programmes has been demonstrated for selected low-risk convalescing CHD patients.[46] The overriding concern here is to ensure that exercise is of only moderate intensity because cardiovascular emergencies are known to be related to inappropriately high exercise intensity, particularly in patients with known myocardial ischaemia during exercise.[47]

Who should receive cardiac rehabilitation? Special needs

Cardiac rehabilitation services were originally designed for patients recovering from an acute MI, and experience is greatest with this group. Those recovering from CABG, percutaneous transluminal coronary angioplasty or stable angina pectoris will also benefit. There is a general perception that post-CABG patients are more stable, and their exercise training may be progressed more rapidly, than post-MI patients or those with chronic stable angina. Chronic heart failure was, until recently, considered an absolute contra-indication to participation in exercise training, but studies have now demonstrated that either walking[48] or home-based exercise on a cycle ergometer[49] can increase exercise tolerance and decrease symptoms in patients with congestive heart failure. Moreover, the very low exercise capacity of these patients means that even small improvements can be important for the activities of daily living.

Older patients previously had less access to rehabilitation. In the UK, for example, data for 1989[42] showed that more than half the programmes had an age limit, usually 65. There has been a progressive increase in the population over 65, with a particularly large increase in those older than 80. In the US, more than one-third of all coronary arteriography, coronary angioplasty, CABG and pacemaker implantation procedures are performed in patients over the age of 65[17] — who now have increasing expectations of resuming a life in which they are reasonably well, alert and active. Amongst older people in particular, decisions about who should receive exercise training will depend on judgements about what constitutes a successful outcome.

Summary

The occurrence of clinical episodes of CHD indicates that patients have accelerated atherosclerosis. If further events are to be averted, progression of atherosclerosis must be slowed or prevented. Exercise has to be *frequent* and *continued* throughout life if it is to contribute to this goal. Early gains in functional capacity developed through hospital-based programmes should not be regarded as an end in themselves, but as a means of achieving a more physically active lifestyle.

Patients with several different manifestations of cardiovascular disease can benefit from exercise rehabilitation, but the prevalence of sedentariness means that many patients have little previous experience of exercise. In England, 70% of men and 80% of women take insufficient exercise to confer health gains.[49] For this reason, and because of the range of differences in pathology, in the total burden of cardiovascular risk, and in current and earlier attitudes towards exercise, an *individual approach* to exercise rehabilitation is indicated. The emphasis needs to be on tailoring the exercise prescription to individual patient needs; this implies that procedures for risk stratification are in place, and that both hospital and home-based programmes can be implemented. These, in turn, depend critically on the availability of trained personnel able to make their specialist input to the whole range of rehabilitation needs of the patient.

A useful set of audit points to assess the success of any exercise programme is given in the Appendix to this chapter.

References

1. Leon AS, Certo C, Comoss P, Franklin BA, *et al.* Position statement of the American Association of Cardiovascular and Pulmonary Rehabilitation. Scientific evidence of the value of cardiac rehabilitation services with emphasis on patients following myocardial infarction. Section 1: Exercise conditioning component. *Journal of Cardiopulmonary Rehabilitation* 1990;**10**:79–87.
2. Saltin B, Rowell LB. Functional adaptations to physical activity and inactivity. *Federation Proceedings* 1980;**39**:1506–13.
3. Wenger NK. Rehabilitation of the patient with coronary heart disease. *Postgraduate Medical Journal* 1989;**85**:369–80.
4. Gollnick PD, Armstrong RB, Saltin B, Saubert CW, *et al.* Effect of training on enzyme activity and fiber composition of human skeletal muscle. *Journal of Applied Physiology* 1973;**34**:107–11.
5. Ingjer F. Effects of endurance training on muscle fibre ATP-ase activity, capillary supply and mitochondrial content in man. *Journal of Physiology* 1979;**294**:419–32.

6. Ehsani AA, Biello DR, Schultz J, Sobell BE, Holloszy JO. Improvement of left ventricular contractile function in patients with coronary artery disease. *Circulation* 1986;**74**:350–8.

7. Todd IC, Ballantyne D. Antianginal efficacy of exercise training: a comparison with β blockade. *British Heart Journal* 1990;**64**:14–9.

8. Todd IC, Ballantyne D. Effect of exercise training on the total ischaemic burden: an assessment by 24 hour ambulatory electrocardiographic monitoring. *British Heart Journal* 1992;**68**:560–6.

9. O'Connor GT, Buring JE, Yusuf S, Goldhaber SZ, *et al.* An overview of randomised trials of rehabilitation with exercise after myocardial infarction. *Circulation* 1989;**80**:234–44.

10. Oldridge NB, Guyatt GH, Fischer MS, Rimm AA. Cardiac rehabilitation after myocardial infarction: combined experience of randomised clinical trials. *Journal of the American Medical Association* 1988;**260**:945–50.

11. Berlin JA, Colditz GA. A meta-analysis of physical activity in the prevention of coronary heart disease. *American Journal of Epidemiology* 1990;**132**:612–28.

12. Shaper G, Wannamethee G. Physical activity and ischaemic heart disease in middle-aged British men. *British Heart Journal* 1991;**66**:384–94.

13. Schuler G, Hambrecht R, Schlierf G, Niebauer J, *et al.* Regular physical exercise and low-fat diet: effects on progression of coronary artery disease. *Circulation* 1992;**86**:1–11.

14. Brown BG, Zhao X-Q, Sacco DE, Alber JJ. Lipid lowering and plaque regression. New insights into prevention of plaque disruption and clinical events in coronary disease. *Circulation* 1993;**87**:1785–91.

15. Haskell WL, Sims C, Myll J, Botz WM, *et al.* Coronary artery size and dilating capacity in ultradistance runners. *Circulation* 1993;**87**:1076–82.

16. Kestin AS, Ellis PA, Barnard MR, Erichetti A, *et al.* Effect of strenuous exercise on platelet activation state and reactivity. *Circulation* 1993;**88**:1502–11.

17. Wenger NK. Rehabilitation of the coronary patient: a preview of tomorrow. *Journal of Cardiopulmonary Rehabilitation* 1991;**11**:93–8.

18. Haskell WL. The influence of exercise training on plasma lipids and lipoproteins in health and disease. *Acta Medica Scandinavica* 1986(Suppl 711):25–37.

19. Hurley BF. Effects of resistance training on lipoprotein profiles: a comparison to aerobic exercise training. *Medicine and Science in Sports and Exercise* 1989;**21**: 689–93.

20. Superko HR. Exercise training, serum lipids and lipoprotein particles: is there a change threshold? *Medicine and Science in Sports and Exercise* 1991;**23**:677–85.

21. Houmard JA, Bruno NJ, Bruner RK, McCammon MR, *et al.* Effects of exercise training on the chemical composition of plasma LDL. *Arteriosclerosis, Thrombosis and Vascular Biology* 1994;**14**:325–30.

22. Morton AR, Stanforth PR, Freund BJ, Joyner MJ, *et al.* Alterations in plasma lipids consequent to endurance training and beta-blockade. *Medicine and Science in Sports and Exercise* 1989;**21**:288–92.

23. Frayn KN. Insulin resistance and lipid metabolism. *Current Opinion in Lipidology* 1993;**4**:197–204.

24. Merrill JR, Holly RG, Anderson RL, Rifai N, *et al.* Hyperlipemic response of young trained and untrained men after a high fat meal. *Arteriosclerosis* 1989;**9**:217–23.

25. Burnstein R, Polychronakos C, Toews CJ, MacDougall JD, *et al.* Acute reversal of the enhanced insulin action in trained athletes: associated with insulin receptor changes. *Diabetes* 1985;**34**:756–6.

26. Mikines KJ, Sonne B, Tronier B, Galbo H. Effects of training and detraining on dose-response relationship between glucose and insulin secretion. *American Journal of Physiology* 1989;**256**:E588–96.

27. Ballor DL, Keesey RE. A meta-analysis of the factors affecting exercise-induced changes in body mass, fat mass and fat-free mass in males and females. *International Journal of Obesity* 1991;**15**:717–26.

28. Arroll B, Beaglehole R. Does physical activity lower blood pressure: a critical review of the clinical trials. *Journal of Clinical Epidemiology* 1992;**45**:439–47.

29. Hagberg JM, Montain SJ, Martin WH, Ehsani AA. Effect of exercise training in 60–69 year old persons with essential hypertension. *American Journal of Cardiology* 1989;**64**:348–53.

30. Cononie CC, Graves JE, Pollock ML, Phillips MI, *et al.* Effect of exercise training on blood pressure in 70 to 79 year old men and women. *Medicine and Science in Sports and Exercise* 1991;**23**:505–11.

31. Richter EA, Turcotte L, Heslep P, Kiens B. Metabolic responses to exercise. Effects of endurance training and implications for diabetes. *Diabetes Care* 1992;**15**(Suppl 4):1767–75.

32. Aldred HE, Hardman AE. Low intensity exercise after consumption of a high fat meal decreases postprandial lipaemia during the recovery period. *Proceedings of the Nutrition Society* 1993;**52**:309.

33. Sady SP, Thompson PD, Cullinane EM, Kantor MA, *et al.* Prolonged exercise augments plasma triglyceride clearance. *Journal of the American Medical Association* 1986;**256**:2552–5.

34. Aldred HE, Perry I, Hardman AE. The effect of a single bout of brisk walking on postprandial lipemia in normolipemic young adults. *Metabolism* 1994;**43**:836–41.

35. Mittleman MA, Maclure M, Tofler GH, Sherwood JB, *et al.* Triggering of acute myocardial infarction by heavy physical exertion — protection against triggering by regular exertion. *New England Journal of Medicine* 1993;**329**:1684–90.

36. Willich SN, Lewis M, Löwel H, Arntz H-R, *et al.* Physical exertion as a trigger of acute myocardial infarction. *New England Journal of Medicine* 1993;**329**:1684–90.

37. Morris JN, Clayton DG, Everitt MG, Semmence AM, Burgess EH. Exercise in leisure time: coronary attack and death rates. *British Heart Journal* 1990;**63**:325–34.

38. Paffenbarger RS, Hyde RT, Wing AL, Hsieh C-C. Physical activity, all-cause mortality, and longevity of college alumni. *New England Journal of Medicine* 1986;**314**:605–13.

39. American College of Sports Medicine. *Guidelines for exercise testing and prescription*, 4th edn. Philadelphia, London: Lea and Febiger, 1991.

40. Vander LB, Franklin BA, Wrisley D, Rubenfire M. Acute cardiovascular responses to nautilus exercise in cardiac patients: implications for exercise training. *Annals of Sports Medicine* 1986;**2**:165–9.

41. Featherstone JF, Holly RG, Amsterdam EA. Physiological responses to weight lifting in coronary artery disease. *American Journal of Cardiology* 1993;**71**:287–92.

42. Horgan J, Bethell H, Carson P, Davidson C, *et al.* Working party on cardiac rehabilitation. *British Heart Journal* 1992;**67**:412–8.

43. Fletcher BJ, Lloyd A, Fletcher GF. Outpatient rehabilitative training in patients with cardiovascular disease: emphasis on training method. *Heart and Lung* 1988;**17**:199–205.

44. Van Camp SP, Peterson RA. Cardiovascular complications of outpatient cardiac rehabilitation programs. *Journal of the American Medical Association* 1986;**256**:1160–3.

45. American College of Cardiology. Recommendations on cardiovascular rehabilitation. *Journal of the American College of Cardiology* 1986;**7**:451–3.

46. DeBusk RF, Haskell WL, Miller NH, Berra K, Taylor CB, in cooperation with Berger WE and Law H. Medically-directed at-home rehabilitation soon after uncomplicated acute myocardial infarction: a new model for patient care. *American Journal of Cardiology* 1985;**55**:251–7.

47. Hassock KF, Hartung R. Cardiac arrest associated with supervised cardiac rehabilitation. *Journal of Cardiac Rehabilitation* 1982;**2**:402–8.

48. Kavanagh T. Exercise and congestive heart failure: the Toronto rehabilitation centre experience. *Canadian Association of Cardiac Rehabilitation* 1993;**2**:10.

49. Coats AJS, Adamopoulos S, Meyer TE, Conway J, Sleight P. Effects of physical training in chronic heart failure. *Lancet* 1990;**335**:63–6.

Appendix

Audit points

- Number attending hospital-based programme
- Number who drop out of hospital-based programme
- Number of women who attend and who drop out
- Number who return to pre-illness physical activity level
- Evaluation of functional capacity prior to exercise prescription
- Home-based programme: prescription and evaluation of compliance
- Training in pulse palpation
- Number developing complications

6 The vocational component

Michael Joy
Consultant Cardiologist, St Peter's Hospital, Chertsey

Stewart Donald
Senior Registrar in Rehabilitation Medicine, Astley Ainslie Hospital, Edinburgh

PART 1: AN OVERVIEW

Michael Joy

Ischaemic heart disease (IHD) (International Classification of Diseases (ICD) 410–414) was the certificated cause of death in almost 150,000 men and women in England and Wales in 1990. Diseases of the circulation (ICD390–459) accounted for nearly half of all deaths. In this cohort, 18,917 males and 5,790 females died of the consequences of coronary heart disease (CHD) before reaching the age of 65 years, the normal age of male retirement in the UK.

Community data from Holland published some 20 years ago suggest that about one-sixth of all patients presenting with IHD do so by way of sudden cardiac death; they will die abruptly without prodromal symptoms which they recognise as premonitory. A fully employed individual spends about one-quarter of his time at work, so such events will be bound to occur in the workplace. Two-fifths of newly presenting IHD will do so as myocardial infarction (MI), and up to one-third of these may die, half within 15 min of the onset of symptoms. The occurrence of such events in the work-place may have safety implications, for example, in the operation of machinery.

Attrition of the employed or potentially employable population by IHD is not restricted to cardiac death alone as a contribution will be made by the coronary syndromes which have a diverse clinical profile. CHD predicts coronary events; a patient in whom coronary atheroma has been identified represents an impaired life in insurance terms, and may be an unattractive proposition to employers, particularly as certain occupations have statutory (ie legally binding) or non-statutory (ie advisory) fitness requirements.

Statutory/non-statutory fitness standards

Certain industries, for example, transportation, have statutory medical fitness requirements which are the subject of local, national or, in the case of aviation, international agreements. An employee in these industries normally has to demonstrate maintenance of the relevant fitness standard as part of his contract of employment. Concern is not restricted only to the safety of the individual but also to the safety of those for whom that individual (eg bus or railway engine driver) is directly or indirectly responsible.

If CHD is suspected or demonstrated, any functional impairment and the likely impact on prognosis must be established. Furthermore, all likely presentations of the coronary syndromes must be taken into account, not only those which may produce an acute and total incapacitation. There is also the possibility of symptoms of sufficient severity with which, while the patient remains conscious, he or she would not be able to function effectively.

Some industries, such as the fire and police services, have non-statutory fitness requirements, and adverse judgements about continuing employability are equally disadvantageous to the individual. Such judgements need to be objective and fair, yet still protect the public. They represent a major challenge to occupational medicine, and there has been an appropriate and increasing interest in their evolution over the past decade.

Recovery and rehabilitation

The past decade has seen an expansion of the cardiological sub-specialty of rehabilitation. It is multidisciplinary, and still sufficiently young for it to be fashionable to define its objectives in any general statement about rehabilitation. Essentially, the aim of rehabilitation is to regain and, if possible, improve the previous physical, social, emotional and occupational status of the individual. A comprehensive approach should start in hospital and involve education about risk factor management, and emotional and psychological support. Exercise training should aim to make good any physiological deficits associated with, and improve the psychological attitude to, the illness. There is some evidence that such an approach may reduce the subsequent event rate and possibly mortality.

The heart and heart work

There has been a striking change in the manual component of work over the past four decades. At the beginning of this period, two-thirds of the population might have been involved in heavy manual work; it is now closer to one-twentieth. Precise data are difficult to obtain about the demands of the workplace upon the cardiovascular system because a number of external influences are at play. These include mental and emotional activity (stress), environmental factors — ambient temperature and noise — as well as the energy expended at work. In general terms, most occupations now require little more work output than normal household activities such as gardening and hoovering. There is thus often little reason for all than the more symptomatic individuals to be considered unfit for non-manual work in industries in which safety is not a critical consideration.

Coronary heart disease and the transportation industries

There are about one million holders of vocational driving licences in the UK and probably 20–24 million holders of current ordinary (Group I) driving licences. Following a recent change in nomenclature, vocational licences are covered by the Group II requirements, which include large goods vehicles and passenger carrying vehicles. Goods vehicles of 7.5 metric tonnes and above require a driver to hold a Group II licence, although under European Union (EU) law this cut-off point may in due course be reduced to 4 metric tonnes. These terms supplant the terms 'heavy goods vehicle' (HGV) and 'public service vehicle' (PSV), respectively. An initial attempt by the EU, in concert with the European Society of Cardiology, to establish a European standard failed, partly because the starting points of the requirements were so different. After a number of meetings, no conclusions were drawn; as a result, the UK went ahead alone and, following a series of meetings by a working group, published a revised standard in September 1993.

The cardiovascular fitness requirements for a Group I licence have always been realistic in the UK, but the same cannot be said of the Group II standards. Specifically, an ordinary driving licence holder is permitted to drive unless there is a relevant disability (eg epilepsy, severe angina provoked by driving). A prospective disability limits the period of validity of the licence, an example of which might be sino-atrial disease. In general, a driver is legally liable to inform the Driver and Vehicle Licensing Authority (DVLA) of such disability, and strongly advised also to inform his insurance company. He is also required to declare himself unfit to drive if he is subject to disabling dizziness or unexplained loss of consciousness.

The requirements for vocational drivers are more coherent and less restrictive than formerly. They are expanded in the DVLA publication, *At a glance guide to current medical standards of fitness to drive.*[1] In determining fitness following the manifestations of CHD, much reliance is placed upon the predictive capability of the exercise electrocardiogram (ECG). In general terms, a driver is required to demonstrate his ability to complete three stages of the Bruce protocol without evidence of myocardial ischaemia. It is appreciated that its predictive powers are limited — but only 0.1% of road traffic accidents are attributable to a medical cause, and only 10–25% of those have a cardiovascular cause. There are some 250,000 notifiable accidents in the UK each year so, at worst, only 25–50 accidents would be attributable to cardiovascular cause, in spite of probable widespread ignorance or avoidance of the relevant requirements.

Aviation

The aviation environment is the only one in which standards of operation and personnel licensing, including medical certification, are agreed by international statute. The responsible agency is the International Civil Aviation Organisation (ICAO), based in Montreal. The ICAO has recently expanded its activities in Europe, together with the EU and others, to set up the European Civil Aviation Conference which will eventually become the greater European regulatory agency (the Joint Aviation Authorities). At present, the Civil Aviation Authority is responsible for all aspects of certification of aircrew, aircraft and airfields in the UK. Much effort has been directed towards examining the cardiological standards of aircrew, notably in the UK. There have now been three workshops on aviation cardiology (two in the UK[2,3] and one European[4]) which have discussed the issues involved. This initiative has recognised the substantial investment in terms of training and experience of an airman, leaving aside the desirability of his rehabilitation in the event of some cardiovascular problem. The latitude which could be taken without prejudicing aviation safety was the focus of much discussion at these workshops and led to the evolution of the so-called 1% rule. (In brief, this rule states that an airman who has a >1% mortality risk per year, with associated morbidity, is unfit to fly.)

In general terms, certification to fly may be granted in best-risk subjects following the discovery of CHD, an MI, coronary surgery and, in a few cases, percutaneous transluminal coronary angioplasty (PTCA).[5] Minor valvular disease may also not be a contraindication to certification, as may best-risk subjects following aortic valve surgery. Such subjects are normally disbarred from single-crew operation in the commercial environment, but such certification in the recreational environment may be permissible (this may reflect the 25-fold worse accident experience in this group).

Sea

Certain aspects of regulation of activity at sea are within the purview of the International Maritime Organisation. Individual nations are nevertheless responsible for standards of construction, maintenance and operation of craft flying their flag. In the UK, these standards are laid down in the Merchant Shipping (Medical Examination) Regulations (1993). Most cardiovascular conditions disbar, in this case as much for the protection of the individual, who may find himself far from skilled medical treatment if it is required, as for the safe operation of the craft. Furthermore, with the smaller, more economical crews presently being employed, the loss of a key crew member may have financial implications in the event of a diversion and possible operational consequences.

The lifeboat service

The lifeboat service in the UK is operated by a charitable foundation, the Royal National Lifeboat Institution, which is concerned with aspects of design, construction, maintenance and operation of lifeboats not already covered by the existing maritime legislation. There are two categories of operation: inshore and offshore. Age limits for service are 45 years and 55 years for inshore and offshore operation, respectively. In general, patients with significant cardiological problems, including CHD, are ineligible for service, but there is a review process which can consider and, if necessary, waive these requirements.

Diving

The standards of professional diving in the British sector of the North Sea are the responsibility of the Health and Safety Executive. The standards for diving inland and elsewhere in the world are laid down by medical advisory committees. There are five categories. Any history of IHD disbars from diving; this applies whether or not the individual has suffered an MI and/or revascularisation of the myocardium. There is a statutory right of appeal. Recreational diving is under the purview of the British Sub-Aqua Club.

Railways

Before the break up of British Rail by the privatisation legislation the application of medical standards of railwaymen in the UK were vested in the Department of Transport. Railwaymen are divided into footplate men, who require an F certificate, and other (safety-related) staff, who require an A certificate. Many rail workers are covered by this, including track staff and some portering staff. Regular medical examinations are required, but the advisory medical standards are unpublished, and the standards themselves do not have statutory authority. Substantial inherent safeguards exist in railway operations, with automatic track signalling and the employment of vigilance devices. Main line trains travelling at less than 110 mph require only one man in the cab, but faster trains require two. The presence of overt or suspected CHD denies certification to operate a locomotive on a main line, but such an individual may find employment on a branch line or in a marshalling yard.

The fire service

The standards for firemen are laid down by the Home Office, and regular medical examinations are required. In general, an established diagnosis of CHD or the presence of other significant cardiology problems is likely to disbar from operation. Drivers of emergency vehicles exceeding 7.5 metric tonnes are also required to fulfil the requirements of the DVLA Group II licence.

Recreational aspects of cardiovascular disease

Numerous pastimes require some sort of medical fitness, including diving, gliding, hang-gliding and microlight flying. The fitness standards for these are the responsibility of the relevant associations; in general, they are lower than those required for private flying unless instructional work is involved.

Motor racing, whether by amateur or professional drivers, requires a Group I licence. A competition licence, which includes a medical declaration, is also required for competitive driving. In general, the medical requirements for a competition licence are likely to be intermediate between the Group I and Group II licences, but this has not yet been agreed. The regulatory body in the UK is the Royal Automobile Club Motor Sports Association; it has its own medical advisory committee, and promulgates its own (national) standards, which are reviewed periodically.

Motor sports may be divided into three types:

- *motor racing*, in which individuals compete against one another, and for which a licence is required, national or international, depending upon the status of the event;

- *motor rallying*, which requires an ordinary driving licence and no special medical examination;

- *speed events*, in which those taking part do not compete directly against one another, also do not require a special medical examination.

Conclusion

A number of vocations, including some not mentioned above (eg offshore oil operations), require medical fitness standards for the protection either of the individual in a hostile environment or of others when the incapacity of the individual may lead to mishap and harm to himself or others. Certain non-vocational and recreational pastimes (eg motor racing, diving) also require a defined standard of fitness. A better understanding in recent years of the natural history and outcome of the more common cardiovascular conditions has led to a more enlightened attitude, helping to maintain employment and economic status.

References

1. Driver and Vehicle Licensing Authority. *At a glance guide to current medical standards of fitness to drive.* Swansea: DVLA, 1993.

2. Joy M, Bennett G. First United Kingdom workshop in aviation cardiology. *European Heart Journal* 1984;**5**(Suppl A):1–163.

3. Joy M, Bennett G. Second United Kingdom workshop in aviation cardiology. *European Heart Journal* 1988;**9**(Suppl G):1–179.

4. Joy M. First European workshop in aviation cardiology. *European Heart Journal* 1992;**13**(Suppl H):1–175.

5. Russell RO, Abi-Mansour P, Wenger NK. Return to work after coronary bypass surgery and percutaneous transluminal coronary angioplasty: issues and potential solutions. *Cardiology* 1986;**73**:306–22.

Recommended reading

1. DeBusk RF. The Stanford University cardiac rehabilitation programme. *Journal of Myocardial Ischaemia* 1990;**2**:28–36.

2.   Hlatky MA, Haney T, Barefoot JC, Califf RM, *et al.* Medical, psychological
      and social correlates of work disability among men with coronary artery
      disease. *American Journal of Cardiology* 1986;**58**:911–5.

3.   Horgan J, Bethell H, Carson P, Davidson C, *et al.* Working party report on
      cardiac rehabilitation. *British Heart Journal* 1992;**67**:412–8.

4.   Joy M. Vocational aspects of coronary artery disease. In: Weatherall DJ,
      Ledingham JCG, Warrell DA (eds). *Oxford textbook of medicine*, 3rd edn.
      Oxford: Oxford University Press, 1986.

5.   Shanfield SB. Return to work after an acute myocardial infarction: a
      review. *Heart and Lung* 1990;**19**:109–17.

6.   Walling A, Tremblay GJ, Jobin J, Charest J, *et al.* Evaluating the rehabil-
      itation potential of a large population of post myocardial infarction
      patients. Adverse prognosis for women. *Journal of Cardiopulmonary
      Rehabilitation* 1988;**8**:99–106.

7.   Wenger NK, Hellerstein HK. *Rehabilitation of the coronary patient*, 3rd edn.
      New York: Churchill Livingstone, 1992.

PART 2: RETURN TO WORK

Stewart Donald

Return to work continues to feature as one of the stated goals of cardiac rehabilitation. Given the perceived importance of being employed in our society, resuming work is seen as a potent symbol of return to normality, and has been used as an easily measured criterion of successful rehabilitation outcome. However, a variety of interrelated factors, including medical, social, demographic and psychological, can determine whether or not an individual returns to work, some of which cannot be influenced by the efforts of rehabilitation. Furthermore, return to work does not necessarily add to the quality of life of patients,[1] especially if the work is physically or emotionally demanding. But if all aspects leading to the enhancement and maintenance of quality of life are perceived as a worthwhile goal of cardiac rehabilitation, a vocational assessment should surely be included. Because of the multifactorial influences on return to work, patients ideally require individualised assessment and guidance — an approach in line with modern cardiac rehabilitation practice. There is an impression that assessment of work issues may be somewhat sporadic, and vocational aspects of cardiac rehabilitation should provide a rich area of audit and research.

Why should vocational issues be considered important?

The simplest answer to this question is that patients themselves consider issues regarding return to work as important. How early return to work could be achieved was found to be one of the main issues raised by patients four weeks after a first MI.[2] A need to know whether work was harmful or beneficial to the heart was also seen as important,[3] and fear of unemployment and loss of earnings was one of the main anxieties of patients just days following an infarct.[4] Work provides the individual with a number of psychosocial and economic advantages; its loss may have a considerable impact, with knock-on effects like loss of income, status, self-esteem, sense of purpose, opportunity to maintain relationships outwith the family, and the development of creative skills. For those with little job satisfaction, however, or who are nearing retirement age, a recent cardiac event may be seen as an opportunity to reappraise the importance of work in their life. In this case, guidance may be needed about the pros and cons of not returning to work. Lastly, the quick return to work of a well rehabilitated individual has advantages to others, including spouses and employers — and indeed the state, through savings on welfare benefits and increased productivity.

What is the incidence of return to work and what factors are important in determining this?

Most of the epidemiological data on return to work are derived from studies on younger employed males following MI or coronary artery bypass graft (CABG) surgery, but information is also available following PTCA, cardiac transplantation and valve surgery. The literature is sparse on return to work of individuals with disabling cardiac syndromes such as angina pectoris or heart failure, perhaps because so few of them are considered for cardiac rehabilitation programmes. Vocational guidance for either the long-term unemployed or the individual capable of voluntary work has received scant attention.

Available studies have shown that the number returning to work, when they do so, and how well they work depend on a wide variety of interrelated factors.[1,5-7] Failure to resume work may be determined by physical variables such as reduced effort tolerance or symptoms, but non-cardiac factors such as age, psychological reaction to the cardiac event, and length of absence from work tend to be more important determinants. Patient and work factors which adversely affect return to work are listed in Tables 1 and 2. In general, a negative influence is associated with older age groups, female sex, length of absence from work, and persisting symptoms. Patients who value their work, have a high level of education and income, and a positive perception of their recovery with reasonable effort tolerance are more likely to return to work.[7] Most socio-demographic factors are unlikely to be influenced by rehabilitation efforts: among the factors amenable to change, psychological factors tend to contribute more to the level of disability of the patient than either medical or physical problems.[8,9]

Myocardial infarction

The return to work rate after MI varies between 62% and 92%.[10-12] The typical duration of absence from work has fallen in recent years and is now about 60–70 days post-infarct.[13-15] Many of those who return to work do not continue for long, with one study showing a drop from 90% initially to 70% by one-year post-infarct.[16] Many

Table 1.
Patient factors adversely determining return to work in cardiac disease.

Demographic:
 OLDER AGE (nearing retirement)
 FEMALE SEX

Medical:
 size of infarct
 number of previous infarcts
 ejection fraction <40%
 persisting symptoms
 EFFORT TOLERANCE
 unpredictable complications (unstable angina, dysrhythmias, syncope)
 coincident chronic disabling disease

Socio-economic:
 LOW EDUCATIONAL LEVEL
 low social class
 LOW INCOME
 high community unemployment level
 favourable insurance/disability income
 favourable pension arrangements for early retirement

Psychological:
 PSYCHOLOGICAL REACTIONS (anxiety, depression)
 personality traits (maladaptive coping strategies, type A behavioural
 patterns)
 PERCEPTION OF THE ILLNESS (knowledge, beliefs, expectations, attributions)
 cognitive functioning (impairments of memory, attention, judgement)
 perceived occupational stresses (heavy work, deadlines, shift work,
 personal relationships, productivity agreements, bonus schemes,
 retraining, travel to and from work)
 reactions and attitudes (of family, employer, colleagues, DOCTOR)

Capitals denote factors having a relatively high negative predictive value.

experience a reduction in workload and working hours, leading to loss of income and job satisfaction[16-20] and, without rehabilitation, less than half work as effectively as before their illness.[4] Patients over age 60 and women are less likely to return to work post-MI. Lower socio-economic status is associated with a delay, and those with physically demanding jobs are particularly less likely to return to or remain at work.

There is a significant relationship between anxiety and depression and return to work. Negative expectations about work closely related to the patients' initial reaction to their illness, particularly if they are depressed or express hopelessness about the future.[21] Insufficient knowledge and wrongly held beliefs are also associated

Table 2.
Work factors adversely determining return to work in cardiac disease.

General:
> nature of work (physical, shift work)
> LENGTH OF ABSENCE FROM WORK
> sporadic work record
> job satisfaction

Statutory limitations:
> train drivers, airline pilots, merchant seafarers, police officers, fire brigade officers, deep sea divers, PSV and HGV drivers

Environmental hazards:
> physically or emotionally demanding
> temperature and pressure stresses
> electromagnetic fields (if fitted with pacemaker)
> exposure to toxic substances (eg carbon monoxide, carbon tetrachloride)

Attitudes:
> employer
> colleagues
> DOCTOR

Capitals denote factors having a relatively high negative predictive value.
HGV = heavy goods vehicle
PSV = public service vehicle

with negative expectations and other forms of maladjustment, leading to failure to return to work.[22] Severe symptoms of angina and shortness of breath following an MI are more likely to lead to reduced return to work rates,[4] as is clinical severity of the infarct in some studies. Generally, however, in those demonstrating a negative association, psychosocial factors are stronger predictors. Most of those who suffer a cardiac arrest return to work unless moderate to severe memory impairment results, when work tends not to be feasible.[23,24]

Coronary artery bypass graft surgery

Despite providing symptomatic relief for over 90% of patients in the initial post-operative years, CABG surgery has proved disappointing in terms of returning people to work,[6] with rates varying from as low as 17% to 85%. In some studies, surgery was no more effective than medical therapy in maintaining continued employment.[6,25,26] Other studies have shown more positive results[27,28] but failure to return to work is largely due to non-medical factors.[26]

One of the strongest predictors for failure to return to work is a prolonged period of absence pre-operatively. Another significant predictor is the patient's pre-operative expectation of resuming employment. Of patients asked whether they felt they would be able to get back to work after their surgery, 82% of those who replied 'yes' did return compared to 40% and 38% of those who said 'no' or were uncertain, respectively.[29] Other important positive predictive factors post-CABG include younger age, relief of symptoms, absence of significant psychological distress, and a positive attitude from medical staff.

Percutaneous transluminal coronary angioplasty

As in CABG surgery, return to work rates after PTCA are higher in those working right up to the time of the procedure (84–100%).[6,30] Important advantages of angioplasty include a rapid return of exercise capability, and thus an earlier return to work. However, most studies have been performed in a highly select group of young males with a low incidence of MI, a short duration of angina, single-vessel disease, and well preserved left ventricular function.

Cardiac transplantation

A survey of seven heart transplant centres in the USA found a return to work rate of 45% following cardiac transplantation. Factors exerting a negative influence include the length of medical disability prior to surgery, the patient's perception of his disability and the loss of disability-related income.[31]

Who needs vocational rehabilitation?

Given the importance and potential source of concern to patients, everybody of employment age who requires cardiac rehabilitation should be offered guidance on return to work. The components of rehabilitation and the degree of emphasis on work issues will vary according to the individual and the perceived importance of the part played by the determining factors (Table 1). It would seem logical that the greater the number or significance of adverse factors with respect to return to work in a given individual, the more input that person may require. This approach depends on a number of issues:

- whether resources are available locally to provide the necessary input;
- how motivated the patient and employer are;
- how modifiable the problems are perceived to be; and
- how proactive the clinician is in targeting such individuals.

If it were left to the patient to seek advice regarding return to work, the inverse care law may apply (ie those most in need of help are least likely to seek it). As for the long-term unemployed and those receiving disability benefits, the poor return to work rates would seem to justify a minimalist approach to vocational guidance, although little can be said because of the relative poverty of research in this group.

What should be the goals of vocational rehabilitation?

The structure and process of any vocational rehabilitation service will realistically depend upon the availability of resources locally as well as on individual patient priorities. To achieve any hope of a successful outcome, the goals of both should approximate as closely as possible. Preservation of quality of life is a universal goal of patients in cardiac rehabilitation,[2] but return to work may not necessarily achieve this.[1] If the patient wishes to return, the goals of a vocational service would be to offer assessment and guidance on:

- whether an individual has the capacity to return to work:
  - physically and psychologically,
  - without incurring risk to themselves,
  - without incurring risk to others;[32]
- how soon a return to work can be achieved;
- once returned to work, how work capacity and job satisfaction can be maintained.

If a patient does not wish to return to work, the efforts of a vocational service should tend towards assessment and guidance on:

- whether the decision is based on a realistic appraisal of his situation;
- if realistic, how the potentially negative effects of unemployment and early retirement can be minimised — this would also apply to those judged incapable of return to work.

How could resources be used to provide vocational rehabilitation?

In general, the skills and equipment should be available in all districts to provide some form of vocational assessment, even without a formal cardiac rehabilitation programme. Utilising the available resources will depend on health professionals taking the initiative in pursuing the issue of return to work with their patients. The appointment of a professional responsible for coordinating rehabilitation has great merits. If access to resources in separate trust hospitals is required, the cooperation of management is essential, with agreed policies on issues of funding and access to avoid delays in providing the service.

It has been recommended that every major district hospital should incorporate a cardiac rehabilitation service,[33] but this has not yet been widely adopted. The key roles in and greatest opportunities for providing vocational rehabilitation will necessarily fall to nursing and medical staff, including general practitioners (GPs), cardiologists, general physicians and cardiac surgeons.

General practitioners

The GP has a pivotal role: he is routinely called upon to judge a patient's fitness to work for the purposes of social security and statutory sick pay, often being in the position of making a decision on empirical grounds without specific guidance from specialist sources. GPs should be encouraged to refer early for a cardiology opinion when they have judged an individual to be unfit for work due to the development of cardiac symptoms. Specific mention should be made in the referral letter of work status and the importance to the individual of return to work.

A patient discharged from hospital following an MI or cardiac surgery will usually visit his GP within the first week for provision of medications and Form Med 3[34] (the statement of advice on refraining from work). This provides an ideal opportunity for the GP to review the issue of return to work by gaining an impression of the patient's attitude to this and to check the patient's understanding of the vocational advice given in hospital. Early signs of an adverse psychological or physical state or of concerns regarding return to work can also be picked up and managed accordingly. It would not be unreasonable for the GP to seek further advice from a cardiologist, liaison psychiatrist, clinical psychologist, occupational health physician or even employer (with the consent of the patient) if the issue remains in doubt. The GP is required to make a judgement on the duration of incapacity and state this on Form Med 3. The decision should be based on the earliest possible occasion that a review assessment is likely to lead to a concrete date of return to work (see under the timing of assessment).

Hospital teams

Hospital teams, with their expertise and resources, are theoretically well placed to make a vocational assessment and judgements on risk stratification and prognosis. Assessment of prognosis and physical capacity with advice tailored to the individual can speed return to work.[35] This has been shown in patients identified as at low risk for cardiac events by demonstrating a well preserved physical capacity and providing explicit advice regarding prognosis, physical capacity and return to work to both the patients and their family practitioners.[36] The key elements of intervention are pre-discharge risk stratification, early exercise testing and explicit medical advice. With respect to CABG surgery, the pre-operative preparation of patient and family by both physician and surgeon, stressing that one of the principle goals of surgery is to return the patient to work — and that this is highly likely to be achieved — has been shown to have a positive effect.[37,38]

Review clinics can be timed to coincide with the earliest occasion that an individual is likely to be considered fit for work, based on risk stratification on discharge. This review provides an opportunity to make a final judgement on fitness for work, with explicit advice given to the patient. If a return to work date is agreed at the review clinic, this information should be communicated to the GP as quickly as possible because he will require time to arrange a review appointment in order to issue the final 'closed' Form Med 3 which states the date of return. In practice, this approach relies on a sufficient appreciation of all the psychological and social factors, and the GP may wish to review arrangements for return to work with the patient and employer. Direct communication with an occupational health physician allied to the place of employment at this stage should help smooth the transition. The value of a further review by the GP or a hospital practitioner once the patient is back at work is uncertain.

The cardiac rehabilitation programme

The effects on return to work rates of participating in a cardiac rehabilitation programme have been equivocal. One comprehensive programme demonstrated a higher maintained work rate at 2–5 years in under-55 year olds.[22] Results of some studies of rehabilitation programmes have been disappointing, but may reflect a lack of attention paid to psychological factors or a failure to adopt a risk stratification approach with vocational assessment and counselling appropriate to the individual. Exercise-based rehabilitation programmes have been shown to improve the rate of return, even in patients belonging to a low social class and having a strenuous job.[39,40]

The role of a cardiac rehabilitation coordinator is emerging as a means of facilitating rehabilitation and is suited to the skills of the nurse specialist in particular. Given the responsibility of liaising with relevant professionals, family and employers, and perhaps training in vocational counselling, more emphasis can be given to vocational issues than currently exists in most programmes. Indeed, a survey of the 91 established outpatient programmes in the UK revealed that only one has a designated vocational counsellor.[33]

No cardiac rehabilitation programme should be without limits, and return to work could be a specified goal. The education component of a programme should cover return to work. This may have limitations in group settings, in which case sessions should be based on a poll of questions commonly raised by patients on the issue of return to work, and dealt with by a professional with some direct experience on the subject.

Specialised work evaluation

Specialised work evaluation may be required where doubts exist as to the capacity of an individual to resume work on either physical or statutory grounds. Referral to an occupational health physician should then be considered, ideally one familiar with the physical requirements of the job. He or she can often provide objective job analysis information on the static/dynamic characteristics of the work, the energy requirements, and environmental and psychological stressors. Liaison with the cardiologist will be necessary as an evaluation may include exercise testing and access to ambulatory equipment for on-the-job studies. Evaluation of the importance of intellectual impairment following cardiac arrest or bypass surgery may require the help of a neuropsychologist. Many occupational therapists have expertise in work-related issues and are a potentially underutilised resource.

How should vocational issues be assessed?

Vocational assessments should be in line with the goals of vocational rehabilitation, and the guidance based on them individualised. However, a useful way of summarising assessments is to place the patient in one of three categories, which may take into account physical, psychological or work-related factors:

1. *Low risk*: return to work can be expected with confidence.

2. *Intermediate risk*: return to work may be possible, but further rehabilitation or evaluation is necessary.

3. *High risk*: return to work is doubtful or not possible.

The timing of assessment

Factors determining viability of return to work can be assessed pre-discharge, and risk stratification made at this stage (Phase I). Rehabilitation and follow-up arrangements after a patient has been discharged following an MI or cardiac surgery may differ. The working party report on cardiac rehabilitation recommended that functional and training assessments be carried out at 6–12 weeks (Phase III).[33] An improvement in functional capacity occurs in most post-infarct patients after one month, and optimum functional capacity may be achieved earlier in those who exercise.[41,42] In uncomplicated post-infarct cases, advice can be given to return to work at 32 days.[36] More specific guidelines for assessing occupational working capacity have been recommended:

- within five weeks for medically uncomplicated MI.

- seven weeks after CABG; and

- one week after successful angioplasty.[43]

It would seem reasonable to use these guidelines as a basis for determining the timing of a medical review, which should have an evaluation of return to work as one of its explicit aims.

The nature of assessment

Cardiac factors. Ideally, a vocational assessment should involve evaluation of all the determinants of return to work but, as time and resources do not permit this counsel of perfection, a minimum standard can be adopted. Routine medical assessment may already have led to reasonable information about mortality risk and functional capacity both from clinical presentation and from investigations as to infarct size and left ventricular function. The exercise ECG has a useful place in risk stratification, especially in identifying patients at the extremes of low and very high risk. A negative exercise ECG can give the physician confidence to prescribe an early return to work and be of great psychological benefit to the patient. An estimate of left ventricular capacity, either clinically or through echocardiography, can also give useful prognostic information, although these methods have not been used widely in assessment of work outcome.[12] The New York Heart Association (NYHA) functional classification has been used as an adjunct to other risk stratification determinants.[44]

Psychosocial factors. Considerations of physical factors alone can lead to inappropriate advice regarding return to work.[36] A minimal assessment of work details and psychological function should be possible. In routine clerking, work details are usually recorded in simple descriptive terms only, but further details about the nature of the job and the patient's feelings towards returning to work may help highlight potential difficulties. A rehabilitation-friendly clerking proforma could be devised to help highlight specific areas of importance and encourage the use of a problem list in cardiology and cardiac surgery units. Such initiatives have already been proposed for the management of stroke.[45]

Psychological assessment should ideally be attempted as early as possible, and monitored at various stages during the rehabilitation process. Anxiety, depression and negative health perceptions are important areas of assessment by nursing, medical and therapy staff. Specifically, expressed hopelessness, passivity, fear and doubt or misconceptions about ability to return to work may be used as cues for further assessment and psychological management. Many of the assessment details can be compiled through patient questionnaires and easily administered screening tools for measuring psychological variables like the Hospital Anxiety and Depression scale.[46] An appreciation of the fears and concerns of the family and employer and their significance to the patients would also be highly valuable.

Specialised assessments. Specialised assessments may be of value if there is any doubt about a patient's capacity to work, but especially in those of intermediate or high risk who want to resume work. Their purpose would be to estimate the probability of an individual experiencing a cardiac event on the job when it would be unlikely otherwise. A standard exercise test does not reflect the cardiovascular response to job conditions such as weight carrying and lifting, working in positions other than upright and in the presence of environmental and psychological stressors.[47] Work simulation or on-site monitoring may be valuable, especially if there is a risk to the public.[43] Close cooperation with occupational physicians and employers would be required. The cost-effectiveness of such an approach is not clear, and more research is required to justify more widespread use.

How should vocational guidance be offered?

After assessment, all patients require guidance on whether and when to return to work. Advice should be as positive, specific and realistic as possible, with areas of uncertainty investigated further, including discussions with employers and occupational health physicians. Vocational counsellors should have sufficient skills and knowledge to appreciate the significance of all assessment variables, and guide accordingly. This role may inevitably fall to medical personnel but, at the very least, all units undertaking rehabilitation of the cardiac patient should agree on whose responsibility it is to provide vocational advice. It is vital that any advice given is communicated to the patient's GP as soon as possible. The need for guidance may not be confined to the patient himself — reassurance of the family and employer may remove unnecessary stress and barriers to return to work.

General guidelines for different risk categories

Physical risk factors

Low risk (NYHA Class I or better; >5 MET on exercise ECG) (1 MET = oxygen consumed by awake individual at rest = 3.5 ml/kg/min). The young, previously fit professional male, following an uncomplicated MI or surgical procedure and with a low risk profile, should be encouraged to return to work at the earliest opportunity:

- 4–6 weeks following an MI,
- 8–10 weeks following surgery, and
- one week following angioplasty.

Difficulty may arise when there are statutory limitations on proscribed vocations, psychological barriers become evident, and/or concerns about the capacity to undertake physical work — although for most jobs this should not be a problem.

Intermediate risk (NYHA Class II; 3–5 MET on exercise ECG). For individuals with medium risk return to work is possible but may be less efficient under certain conditions. If this is considered a problem, the following options may apply, for all of which close liaison with the employer would be an advantage:

- modification of the work required to reduce the demands by altering the environment or changing job;

- selective placement in a job with lesser demands;

- vocational training for a job with less energy demands;

- enhancing work capacity by exercise training, psychological support and medical therapy;

- retirement/unemployment.

High risk (NYHA Class III; 2–3 MET on exercise ECG). Part-time or sedentary work is possible, although return to work may depend on close examination of the five options listed for medium-risk individuals.

Very high risk (NYHA Class IV; <2 MET on exercise ECG). Unemployment or retirement is strongly advised. These individuals are functionally too incapacitated to work and are at risk of sudden cardiac events.

Psychological risk factors

If style of work and psychological attitudes are assessed as preventing return to work, further psychological counselling or cognitive behavioural training may be required. The secondary prevention aspect of comprehensive programmes should include training in adapting an individual's approach to work away from type A characteristics. Any misconceptions regarding possible harm at work that continue to prevail should be corrected as confidently as possible by a physician who knows the patient's risk status. The need for clinical psychologist or psychiatric support should be judged according to the individual situation. Once the patient has returned to work, there should be follow-up to support the patient through a potentially anxious initial phase and to screen for adverse reactions. A risk stratification for psychological risk at work is required.

Guidance for those unable to return to work

The loss of work due to redundancy, prohibition by statute or incapacity may cause distress and financial hardship. Vocational counselling should include support and assistance in efforts to find alternative employment or to minimise the potential handicap caused by unemployment. For those considering early retirement, a non-directive approach to counselling to facilitate an informed decision may be preferable.

Reducing duration of absence from work

Those adjudged unfit for work because of symptoms may be at special disadvantage if their symptoms remain uncontrolled for greater than six months. The rehabilitation of patients with angina or heart failure needs wider recognition and research; management needs to work in partnership with medical and surgical teams to reduce waiting list times for cardiac surgery; and GPs, cardiologists, occupational physicians and doctors from the Benefits Agency Medical Service (BAMS) need to collaborate to facilitate the process of return to work.

Summary

Despite return to work being an explicit goal of cardiac rehabilitation, the role of vocational rehabilitation has not received wide recognition. The vocational process aims to achieve an early return to work in a person who is capable, relaxed, confident and content at work. Those who are unable to return can be helped to minimise the disadvantages of unemployment. Even if formal rehabilitation programmes are not locally available, the means to make a reasonable vocational assessment and to give vocational advice are usually accessible. In all cases, good practice depends on the coordination of available resources and the designation of a professional with the relevant skills with a mandate to do this. Medical staff should be pro-active, aiming to give clear explicit advice on return to work whenever possible. More research is required to determine optimal delivery of a vocational rehabilitation service for cardiac patients.

Summary of recommendations

1. Vocational guidance should be available to all with cardiac disease, and form part of a comprehensive cardiac rehabilitation programme.

2. One of the goals of cardiac rehabilitation is to help optimise the conditions to facilitate an appropriate and realistic decision about returning to work.

3. Specific goals of vocational rehabilitation include enabling an early return to work, minimising the conditions which will reduce work capacity, job satisfaction and the adverse effects of unemployment.

4. Vocational guidance should be individualised and based on a full understanding of the clinical, psychological, socio-economic and environmental issues involved for a given patient. Key assessments include risk stratification, job analysis and psychological screening.

5. There should be an early attempt to assess the psychological reactions of the patient. Key areas include evaluation of depression and expressed hopelessness about the future, belief about health status, and expectations of return to work. A useful screening question would be 'how do you feel about going back to work?'

6. One explicit aim of the medical/surgical outpatient or GP review following MI or cardiac surgery should be to assess and advise on return to work. The timing of this review should be at 4–8 weeks, with exercise testing carried out at this stage to assess functional capacity, if considered appropriate. Early exercise testing has a high negative predictive accuracy: a negative test allows the physician to make a confident prediction about return to work.

7. Vocational advice should be given as early as possible to avoid unnecessary anxieties about return to work and to prevent invalidism.

8. Vocational advice should not be conflicting. Those under-taking it should communicate with everyone (above all, the GP) involved in the care of the patient with cardiac disease to encourage a consistent approach and reinforcement of advice. It should be agreed locally by hospital clinicians *who* should give vocational guidance. There is a potential key role here for the cardiac rehabilitation coordinator in facilitating and communicating vocational guidance to all interested parties.

9. Vocational advice should be positive, specific and realistic. If advice depends on further evaluation, this should be arranged as soon as practicable.

10. For some patients, the emphasis on vocational counselling should be to enable the individual to make an informed decision on whether return to work will be of overall benefit to his quality of life.

11. Absence from work should be kept to a minimum duration. This means shortening waiting times for those undergoing CABG surgery, optimising medical treatment, and encouraging a quick return to work if possible.

12. More effort is needed to rehabilitate the patient with disabling angina or cardiac failure, even if he is waiting for a definitive surgical procedure.

13. Vocational aspects of cardiac disease should form part of the higher specialist training in cardiology, rehabilitation medicine and occupational medicine. In-service training on vocational issues should be made available to nurses and therapists involved in cardiac rehabilitation teams.

14. Better links with government agencies should be formed to maintain at work the individual with disabling cardiac disease. Awareness of the important roles of the Department of Employment's placement and assessment counselling team, BAMS, the Chief Scientist's Office, disability research funding, and other statutory agencies like the DVLA may lead to increased opportunities.

15. More research is needed to determine how to optimise delivery of a vocational rehabilitation service, and to evaluate the role and cost-effectiveness of specialist work assessments.

References

1. Mayou R, Bryant B. Quality of life after coronary artery surgery. *Quarterly Journal of Medicine* 1987;**62**:239–45.

2. Cay EL. Psychological aspects of cardiac rehabilitation. *Update* March 1986:377–86.

3. Orzeck SA. Comparison of patients and spouses: needs during the post hospital convalescence phase of myocardial infarction. *Journal of Cardiopulmonary Rehabilitation* 1987;**7**:59–65.

4. Cay EL, Vetter N, Philips A, Dugard P. Return to work after a heart attack. *Journal of Psychosomatic Research* 1973;**17**:231–43.

5. Stewart MJ, Gregor FM. Early discharge and return to work following myocardial infarction. *Social Science and Medicine* 1984;**18**:1027–36.

6. Russell RO, Abi-Mansour P, Wenger NK. Return to work after coronary artery bypass surgery and percutaneous transluminal angioplasty: issues and potential solutions. *Cardiology* 1986;**73**:306–22.

7. Denolin H, Feruglio GA, Gobbato F, Maisano G. Guidelines for return to work after myocardial infarction and/or revascularisation. *European Heart Journal* 1988;**9**(Suppl L):130–1.

8. Wynn A. Unwarranted emotional distress in men with ischaemic heart disease. *Medical Journal of Australia* 1967;**2**:251–87.

9. Nagle R. Factors influencing return to work after myocardial infarction. *Lancet* 1971;**ii**:454–6.

10. Wiklund I, Sanne H, Vedin I, Wilhelmson C. Coping with myocardial infarction: a model with clinical applications, a literature review. *International Rehabilitation Medicine* 1985;**7**:167–75.

11. Smith GR, O'Rourke DF. Return to work after myocardial infarction: a test of multiple hypotheses. *Journal of the American Medical Association* 1988;**259**:1673–7.

12. Shanfield SB. Return to work after an acute myocardial infarction: a review. *Heart and Lung* 1990;**19**:109–17.

13. Hlatky MA, Cotugno HE, Mark DB, O'Connor C, *et al.* Trends in physician management of uncomplicated acute myocardial infarction, 1970–1987. *American Journal of Cardiology* 1988;**61**:515–8.

14. Burgess AW, Lerner DJ, D'Agostino RB. A randomised controlled trial of cardiac rehabilitation. *Social Science and Medicine* 1987;**24**:359–70.

15. Vuopla V. Resumption of work after myocardial infarction in Northern Finland. *Acta Medica Scandinavica* 1986;**530**(Suppl):3–53.

16. Mayou R, Foster A, Williamson B. Psychosocial adjustments in patients one year after myocardial infarction. *Journal of Psychosomatic Research* 1978;**22**:447–53.

17. Doehrman SR. Psychosocial aspects of recovery from coronary heart disease: a review. *Social Science and Medicine* 1977;**11**:199–218.

18. Wiklund I, Sanne H, Wedin A, Wilhelmsson C. Determinants of return to work one year after a first myocardial infarction. *Journal of Cardiac Rehabilitation* 1985;**5**:62–72.

19. Maeland JG, Havik OE. Return to work after a myocardial infarction: the influence of background factors, work characteristics and illness severity. *Scandinavian Journal of Social Medicine* 1986;**24**:183–95.

20. Garrity TF. Vocational adjustment after the myocardial infarction: comparative assessment of several variables suggested in the literature. *Social Science and Medicine* 1973;**7**:705–7.

21. Maeland JG, Havik OE. Psychological predictors for return to work after a myocardial infarction. *Journal of Psychosomatic Research* 1987;**31**:471–81.

22. Hedback B, Perk J. Five year result of a comprehensive rehabilitation programme after myocardial infarction. *European Heart Journal* 1987;**8**:234–42.

23. Eisenberg MS, Hallstrom A, Bergner L. Long term survival after out of hospital cardiac arrest. *New England Journal of Medicine* 1982;**306**:1340–3.

24. Moller M, Holm B, Sindrup A. Electroencephalographic prediction of anoxic brain damage after resuscitation from cardiac arrest in patients with acute myocardial infarction. *Acta Medica Scandinavica* 1978;**203**:31–7.

25. Russell RO, Wayne JB, Kronfeld J, Charles ED, *et al.* Surgical versus medical therapy for treatment of unstable angina: changes in work status and family income. *American Journal of Cardiology* 1980;**45**:134–40.

26. Hammermeister KE, De Rouen TA, English MT, Dodge HT. Effect of surgical versus medical therapy on return to work in patients with coronary artery disease. *American Journal of Cardiology* 1979;**44**:105–11.

27. Wallwork J, Potter B, Caves PK. Return to work after coronary artery surgery for angina. *British Medical Journal* 1978;**ii**:1680–1.

28. Westaby S, Sapsford RN, Bentall HH. Return to work and quality of life after surgery for coronary artery disease. *British Medical Journal* 1979;**ii**:1028–31.

29. Stanton B-A, Jenkins CD, Denlinger P, Savageau JA, *et al.* Prediction of employment status after cardiac surgery. *Journal of the American Medical Association* 1983;**249**:907–11.

30. Holmes DR, Van Raden MJ, Reeder GS, Vlietstra RE. Return to work after coronary angioplasty: a report from the National Heart, Lung and Blood Institute PTCA registry. *American Journal of Cardiology* 1984;**53**:48c–51c.

31. Meister ND, McAleer MJ, Meister JS, Riley JE, *et al.* Returning to work after heart transplantation. *Journal of Heart Transplantation* 1986;**5**:154–61.

32. Pryor DB, Bruce RA, Chaitman BR, Fisher L, *et al.* Task force I: determination of prognosis in patients with ischaemic heart disease. *Journal of the American College of Cardiology* 1989;**14**:1016–25.

33. Horgan J, Bethell H, Carson P, Davidson P, *et al.* Working party report on cardiac rehabilitation. *British Heart Journal* 1992;**67**:412–8.

34. Department of Social Security. *Medical evidence for statutory sick pay, statutory maternity pay and social security incapacity benefit purposes: a guide for registered medical practitioners*; IB 204. Revised, with effect from 13 April 1995.

35. Picard MH, Dennis C, Schwartz RG, Ahn DK, *et al.* Cost benefit analysis of early return to work after uncomplicated acute myocardial infarction. *American Journal of Cardiology* 1989;**63**:1308–14.

36. Dennis C, Houston-Miller N, Schwartz RG, Ahn DK, *et al.* Early return to work after uncomplicated myocardial infarction. *Journal of the American Medical Association* 1988;**260**:214–20.

37. Oberman AL, Wayne JB, Kouchouka NT, Charles ED. Coronary employment status after artery bypass surgery. *Circulation* 1982; **65**(Suppl II):115–9.

38. Liddle NV, Jensen R, Clayton PD. The rehabilitation of coronary surgical patients. *Annals of Thoracic Surgery* 1982;**34**:374–82.

39. Velasco JA, Tormo V, Ridocci F, Grima A. From Spain: return to work after a comprehensive cardiac rehabilitation programme. *Journal of Cardiac Rehabilitation* 1983;**3**:725–8.

40. Boudrez H, De Backer G, Comhaire B. Return to work after myocardial infarction: results of a longitudinal population based study. *European Heart Journal* 1994;**15**:32–6.

41. Wohl A, Lewis H, Campbell W. Cardiovascular function during early recovery from acute myocardial infarction. *Circulation* 1977;**56**:931–7.

42. Hung J, Gordon EP, Houston N, Haskell WL, *et al.* Changes in rest and exercise myocardial perfusion and left ventricular function 3 to 26 weeks after clinically uncomplicated acute myocardial infarction: effect of exercise training. *American Journal of Cardiology* 1984;**54**:943–50.

43. Haskell WL, Brachfeld N, Bruce RA, Davis PO, *et al.* Task force II: determination of occupational working capacity in patients with ischaemic heart disease. *Journal of the American College of Cardiology* 1989;**14**:1025–34.

44. DeBusk RF. The Stanford University cardiac rehabilitation programme. *Journal of Myocardial Ischaemia* 1990;**2**:28–36.

45. Royal College of Physicians of London. *Stroke audit package.* London: RCP, 1994.

46. Zigmond AS, Snaith RP. The hospital anxiety and depression scale. *Acta Psychiatrica Scandinavica* 1983;**67**:361–70.

47. Landes J, Rod JL. Return to work evaluation after coronary events: special emphasis on simulated work activity. *Sports Medicine* 1992;**13**:365–75.

Appendix 1

Audit points

Structure:

- access to vocational counsellor
- access to occupational physician
- access to exercise testing facilities/ambulatory monitor
- existing policy on return to work

Process:

- number of patients expressing problems with return to work

- number offered specific vocational counselling

- documented assessment of work factors

- documented vocational advice (inpatient/outpatient)

- work status noted at hospital outpatient clinics

- return to work covered in education sessions, and patient satisfaction with this

- documented psychological assessment in cardiology/cardiac surgery medical and nursing notes

- communication with GPs on work related issues

- documented spouse's feelings about return to work

- GP follow-up and recorded discussion about return to work

- efforts to help those unable to work gain financial security

Outcome:

- number returning to work, and when

- age and number still at work after 1, 2, 5 and 10 years

- number of women returning to work

- job satisfaction on return to work

- number able to maintain same workload as prior to cardiac event

- number returning to different jobs with same employer

- number needing to reduce to part-time work

- loss of income on return

- perceived loss of status on return

- perceived loss of promotion prospects on return

- outcome in those told positively pre-revascularisation procedure by physician or surgeon that they will be able to return to work

- return to work in those already considering early retirement

Appendix 2

Research

- attributions of work-related factors post-myocardial infarction and their influence on return to work

- early intervention and individualised vocational counselling in high-risk patients

- influence of cognitive behavioural training programmes on return to work

- poll of employers' attitudes and knowledge regarding cardiac disease

- epidemiology studies on return to work and physically demanding jobs

- epidemiology studies on return to work and low socio-economic class

- pre-discharge assessment of job satisfaction and return to work

- measurement of quality of life in those deciding to take early retirement

- evaluation of the role of rehabilitation coordinator and return to work

- use of functional assessment measures in determining work outcome

- use of telemetry/ambulatory monitoring in physically demanding jobs

- evaluation of METs required for specific jobs

- evaluation of return to work as a risk factor in physically demanding jobs

- validation of questionnaires relating to psychological function with respect to return to work

- development of risk assessment profile for failure to return to work

- development of assessments of job satisfaction and work efficiency

- cognitive impairment post-CABG and return to work

- survey of work-related problems reported by patients on their return to work

- stratification of importance of return to work compared with other goals of rehabilitation by professionals involved in cardiac care, including GPs.

- studies on simulated work activity, and return to work rates, psychological variables, validity testing compared with work-place performance and criteria/indications for use.

- validity and reliability of perceived exertion as self-assessment tool during heavy work

- evaluation of the role of exercise testing and NYHA functional classification in return to work

7 The economic component

Alastair Gray

Director, Health Economics Research Centre, Institute of Health Sciences at Wolfson College, Oxford

Heart disease imposes enormous costs on individuals, the National Health Service (NHS) and society in the UK each year, the annual cost to the NHS alone being estimated at £668 million (1992 prices).[1] When scarce health care resources are committed to treating heart disease, and to specific interventions such as cardiac rehabilitation, it is appropriate systematically to evaluate the economic benefits as well as the clinical benefits.

In the USA, it has been estimated that 10–15% of the one million people who survive an acute myocardial infarction (AMI) each year will receive supervised cardiac rehabilitation in an outpatient setting, at an annual gross cost of US$160–240 million.[2,3] At present, little is known about the economic magnitude of cardiac rehabilitation in the UK, although it has been estimated that fewer than half the health districts in the British Isles have an established rehabilitation programme. It has been recommended that every major district hospital treating patients with heart disease should provide a cardiac rehabilitation service;[4] in view of this, information on the cost-effectiveness of cardiac rehabilitation is particularly needed.

Economic evaluation

Economic evaluation involves a family of different techniques.

Cost analysis

The primary concern of cost analysis is to identify the costs associated with a particular activity. The perspective from which the analysis is performed may be relevant to the results. A cost study of a cardiac rehabilitation programme may:

- consider only the direct costs incurred by the health service, and ignore any other costs;
- include costs incurred by patients, for example, out-of-pocket

expenses associated with travel or time off work when they attend a rehabilitation session; or

- add in the costs of equipment, such as exercise bicycles, shoes and clothing recommended as part of the programme.

There is also the perspective of society as a whole. If an effective rehabilitation programme enables patients to return to work more rapidly than without such a programme, society may avoid the costs of reduced output, higher welfare payments and lower tax receipts.

Cost-effectiveness

Studies of cost-effectiveness are concerned to calculate the ratio of the net change in costs to the net change in health outcomes of alternative courses of action.[5] The outcomes may be measured in terms of natural units, such as change in blood pressure, MIs averted, or life-years gained.

Cost utility

In many circumstances, however, possibly including cardiac rehabilitation, an outcome measure such as life-years gained is inadequate as it contains no measure of health-related quality of life. Cost-utility analysis is a procedure which overcomes this problem by measuring outcomes in terms of a composite of quantity and quality of life: quality-adjusted life-years (QALYs).

In considering the results of cost-effectiveness and cost-utility studies, it is important to bear in mind the precise comparison being made. For example, a comparison of cardiac rehabilitation with no rehabilitation will give different results to a comparison of intensive inpatient versus outpatient rehabilitation.

Similarly, it is important to note how the intervention has been defined. Dennis[6] has suggested that comprehensive cardiac rehabilitation services may be considered, from the perspective of the economic analyst, as including any of the following components:

- exercise training and physical reconditioning,
- education and counselling,
- occupational work evaluation,
- diet and drug treatment of hypercholesterolaemia, and
- smoking cessation.

Each of these components may in turn have significant differences. For example, exercise training may or may not involve electrocardiographic (ECG) monitoring equipment and trained medical supervision. The precise content of the intervention will affect an economic analysis at least as much as it would affect a clinical analysis of effectiveness.

Cost studies

Costs of rehabilitation

Estimates of the direct costs of a cardiac rehabilitation programme depend on the type of programme and the setting. For example, the US model of cardiac rehabilitation most often involves up to three sessions per week of exercise training and education for approximately 12 weeks, at a cost of US$65–125 per session (1990 prices). This includes only direct health service costs, and is equivalent to a total cost of US$2,340–6,840, or approximately £750–2,196 (non-sterling costs have been converted into sterling using exchange rates adjusted for purchasing power parity). A detailed model of coronary heart disease in the US, which incorporates a range of prices relating to AMI, suggests a cost of US$2,430 (approximately £780) per patient (1986 prices).[2]

Community-based programmes supervised by physical educators, but without ECG monitoring or the presence of physicians or nurses, have been described in an American context with running costs of less than US$500 per person per year,[7] but the comparative effectiveness of these programmes has not been assessed in a controlled trial. Other American studies have quoted costs midway within the range given above. Ades *et al*,[8] for example, suggest a figure of US$1,152 (£370) for a cardiac rehabilitation programme consisting of three one-hour sessions per week for 12 weeks of aerobic exercise, plus one hour per week of teaching on stress management, diet, cardiac risk factors, symptoms and medication at US$32 (£10) per session (1990 prices).

In Sweden, Levin *et al*[9] estimated a figure of SKr2,743 (£251) per patient (1990 prices) for a rehabilitation programme of two 45-min training sessions a week over three months. In the UK, a working party on cardiac rehabilitation services estimated that the costs of a rehabilitation session varied between £4 and £15 per patient per session, but no details of these estimates were published.[4] Also in the UK, Lewin *et al*[10] attached a cost of £30–50 to a home-based self-help rehabilitation programme consisting of a manual-based course of education, tape-based relaxation and stress management, with some time from a facilitator, but again details of the costings were not published. Accounts from individual UK cardiac rehabilitation units suggest that the average cost per case is in the region of £200 per year, depending on the level of staffing, equipment, and number of sessions in a rehabilitation course.[11] More recently, Gray *et al*[12] have reported that the cost per patient completing a rehabilitation course averaged £370 (1994 prices) in a sample of 16 centres in England and Wales.

Finally, Oldridge *et al*[3] examined a Canadian cardiac rehabilitation programme consisting of a two-session per week, eight-week programme of supervised exercise together with group behavioural and risk factor management. The direct costs per patient were estimated at Can$570 (1987 prices), with a possible range of Can$310–1,050 (approximately £155–525).

Effect of cardiac rehabilitation on hospitalisation costs

If cardiac rehabilitation is effective in reducing cardiac morbidity following MI, it would be anticipated that hospitalisation costs associated with cardiac hospitalisation would be lowered. Ades *et al*[8] examined this in a non-randomised study of 580 patients who had survived an AMI or coronary artery bypass graft (CABG) surgery; 230 of these patients elected to enter a cardiac rehabilitation programme, consisting of a three-month, four-hour per week programme of exercise and risk factor teaching. Interpretation of the results from this study is complicated by baseline differences between the two groups, the non-randomised selection method, variable follow-up periods, and drop-outs from the rehabilitation programme. Over a mean follow-up period of 21 months, the main result was a reduction in hospitalisation costs by US$739 (£237) per patient entering the rehabilitation programme. If physician costs were included, this figure was raised to US$850–887. The cost of providing the rehabilitation programme was US$1,152 (£370) per patient, excluding any travel time or other costs incurred by the patients, so the rehabilitation programme did not yield any savings in direct health care costs.

The Swedish study by Levin *et al*[9] reported a more favourable result. In a five-year follow-up period, rehospitalisation costs were equivalent to a reduction of £786 per patient (1990 prices) in the intervention group compared with the control group, primarily due to shorter lengths of stay rather than to lower admission rates. In comparison, the direct health costs of the rehabilitation programme were equivalent to £251 per patient; a further £270 per patient incurred in out-of-pocket expenses by the patients brought the total cost to £572.

Health service utilisation was measured over a 12-month follow-up period in a Canadian randomised controlled trial of 201 patients after AMI who had mild or moderate anxiety, depression, or both.[3] There were no significant differences between the intervention and control groups in physician utilisation rates, emergency admissions, inpatient days or prescribed medications, but the rehabilitation group made significantly less use of community cardiac rehabilitation services following the intervention.

Finally, a randomised control trial by Lewin *et al*[10] of 176 patients allocated to either a standard package of care or a home-based self-help rehabilitation programme following MI found that significantly more patients in the control group were admitted to hospital in the six months post-MI, but at 12 months the difference was non-significant.

Summarising these studies, there is some evidence — though not in a controlled trial setting — that cardiac rehabilitation may reduce subsequent hospitalisation costs. In so far as any such savings exist, however, they seem to be of about the same magnitude as the costs to the health care system of the rehabilitation programme.

Return to work

A number of studies have considered the impact of cardiac rehabilitation programmes on return to work, but seldom within the framework of a formal economic evaluation. The Swedish five-year follow-up study[9] comparing a cardiac rehabilitation programme (consisting of follow-up at a post-MI clinic, health education and physical training in outpatient groups) with standard care after MI found a significant difference in return to work. Five years after MI, 52% of patients in the intervention group were in active employment compared to 27% of patients in the control group ($p < 0.01$). As a result, production losses due to sick leave and early retirement averaged £47,092 per patient (1990 prices) in the control group, but only £40,615 in the intervention group. This gain of £6,477 was substantially in excess of the £510 cost per patient associated with the rehabilitation programme. The beneficiaries were the patients and the Swedish government exchequer rather than the health service. A 10-year follow-up of the same patients[13] indicated a continuing gain: 59% of patients in the intervention group who had not yet reached retirement age were still in employment versus 22% in the control group ($p < 0.05$).

A randomised controlled trial of work evaluated and of advice by primary physicians also claimed a significant reduction in return to work time: 51 days after uncomplicated MI in the intervention group compared with 75 days in the control group.[14] The cost of the intervention in this US study was placed at US$500 (£160) (1986 prices), with an average increase in earnings of US$2,100 (£674). Improved return to work rates following rehabilitation was also shown in a controlled trial by Bertie *et al.*[15]

Less impressive results were obtained by Perk *et al*[16] in a case-control study of the effects of cardiac rehabilitation after CABG. There was no evidence at one-year or at a 38-month follow-up of a higher rate of return to work in the intervention group. This finding reflects the results obtained by a number of controlled trials of exercise- and advice-based rehabilitation programmes following MI or coronary artery surgery which have not found evidence of improved return to work rates.[17]

Cost-effectiveness studies

The only full cost-effectiveness study of cardiac rehabilitation is the Canadian study by Oldridge *et al*,[3] based on a randomised controlled trial of 210 patients with AMI and mild to moderate anxiety or depression. There was no difference in mortality during a 12-month follow-up; consequently, the trial results were unable to support any calculations of cost per life-year gained.

Using the results from a meta-analysis of cardiac rehabilitation which found significantly less mortality over a three-year period with rehabilitation compared with control patients,[18] Oldridge *et al*[3] estimated a life-year gain per patient of 0.022 (= 8 days) in the three years after the intervention. Taking account of all costs and savings associated with the intervention, this is equivalent to US$21,800 per life-year gained. As Table 1 demonstrates, this gain does not compare favourably with other interventions such as smoking cessation advice, aspirin for all AMIs, beta-adrenergic antagonist therapy for 55 year old high-risk men (see also Olsson *et al*[19]), or even with some categories of cholesterol-lowering or anti-hypertensive therapies, although it is significantly more cost-effective than, for example, captopril or colestipol.

Cost-utility studies

As noted earlier, a potential shortcoming of cost-effectiveness studies is that they do not incorporate any health-related quality-of-life

Table 1.
Cost-effectiveness of cardiac rehabilitation and other interventions.

Intervention	Cost per life-year gained (1991 US$)
Cardiac rehabilitation[3]	21,800
Brief smoking advice during office visit (55 year old men):	
2.7% cessation, 10% relapse[20]	1,200
1% cessation, 50% relapse[20]	9,500
Aspirin for all AMI[21]	3,100
Beta-adrenergic antagonist therapy	
(55 year old high-risk men)[22]	5,300
Monotherapies for hypertension (>94 mmHg):	
Propranolol hydrochloride[23]	1,600
Captopril[23]	106,900
Hypercholesterolaemia (>272 mg/dl):	
Lovastatin (40 mg/day)[24]	17,000
Lovastatin (80 mg/day)[24]	73,000
Hypercholesterolaemia (>265 mg/dl):	
Colestipol (bulk price)[25]	104,500

Table adapted from Reference 3.
AMI = acute myocardial infarction

changes in their measure of outcome. Only one such cost-utility study of cardiac rehabilitation has been performed, again by Oldridge *et al*.[3] Patients in each arm of the trial were asked to score their health status at two, four, eight and 12 months using a time trade-off procedure. These scores were then converted into QALYs. The result was a gain of 0.052 QALYs per patient (= 19 days) among patients in the rehabilitation group compared with the control group in the year after the rehabilitation intervention. This is equivalent to US$9,200 per QALY (95% confidence intervals: US$4,400–24,600), which compares reasonably favourably to other heart disease interventions listed in Table 2. If the assumed mortality benefit, as indicated in the overview by O'Connor *et al*[18], is added into the result, the cost per QALY falls to US$6,800, as also shown in Table 2.

Summary

Knowledge of the economics of cardiac rehabilitation remains sparse, and the few economic evaluations which have been performed are Scandinavian or North American. Precise UK data on

Tablu 2.
Cost utility of cardiac rehabilitation and other interventions.

Intervention	Cost per QALY (1991 US$)
Cardiac rehabilitation:	
12-month follow-up[3]	9,200
36-month benefit[3]	6,800
CABG:	
Left main disease[26]	7,900
1-vessel disease, mild angina[26]	68,200
Diastolic hypertension in 40 year old men:	
Severe (>104 mmHg)[26]	17,700
Mild (95–104 mmHg)[26]	35,900

Table adapted from Reference 3.
CABG = coronary artery bypass graft
QALY = quality-adjusted life year

the content and direct costs of cardiac rehabilitation programmes are a necessary first step before generalising the results of economic evaluations from other countries. The evidence that rehabilitation programmes reduce subsequent health care utilisation and costs is not strong. The only cost-effectiveness study performed so far found no within-trial survival benefit from cardiac rehabilitation. A cost-utility analysis found a small but significant gain in quality of life amongst individuals who had participated in a rehabilitation programme. Overall, the cost-effectiveness of cardiac rehabilitation appears to place it in the middle of the range of heart interventions for which cost-effectiveness data are available, but the lack of firm outcome data means that any such cost-effectiveness estimates must be placed within wide confidence limits.

References

1. Wells N. *Coronary heart disease: the need for action.* London: Office of Health, London, 1987.

2. Wittell EH, Hay JW, Gotto AM. Medical costs of coronary artery disease in the United States. *American Journal of Cardiology* 1990;**65**:432–40.

3. Oldridge N, Furlong W, Feeny D, Torrance G, *et al.* Economic evaluation of cardiac rehabilitation soon after acute myocardial infarction. *American Journal of Cardiology* 1993;**72**:154–61.

4. Horgan J, Bethell H, Carson P, Davidson C, *et al.* Working party report on cardiac rehabilitation. *British Heart Journal* 1992;**67**:412–8.

5. Weinstein MC, Stason WB. Foundation of cost-effectiveness analysis for health and medical practices. *New England Journal of Medicine* 1977; **296**:716–21.

6. Dennis C. Cost-effectiveness in cardiac rehabilitation. *Journal of Cardiopulmonary Rehabilitation* 1991;**11**:128–31.

7. Zohman LR, DiMattai D, Peimer L. Twenty-five years of inexpensive community-based cardiac rehabilitation. *Coronary Artery Disease* 1991;**2**: 409–14.

8. Ades PA, Huang D, Weaver SO. Cardiac rehabilitation participation predicts lower rehospitalization costs. *American Heart Journal* 1992;**123**: 916–21.

9. Levin LA, Perk J, Hedback B. Cardiac rehabilitation — a cost analysis. *Journal of Internal Medicine* 1991;**230**:427–34.

10. Lewin B, Robertson IH, Cay EL, Irving JB, Campbell M. Effects of self-help post-myocardial infarction rehabilitation on psychological adjustment and use of health services. *Lancet* 1992;**339**:1036–40.

11. Turner S. *Basingstoke and Alton cardiac rehabilitation unit: annual report 1993.* Alton, Hants: Alton Health Centre, 1993.

12. Gray AM, Bowman GS, Thompson DR. The cost of cardiac rehabilitation services in England. *Journal of the Royal College of Physicians of London* 1997;**31**:57–61.

13. Hedback B, Perk J, Wodlin P. Long-term reduction of cardiac mortality after myocardial infarction: 10-year results of a comprehensive rehabilitation programme. *European Heart Journal* 1993;**14**:831–5.

14. Dennis C, Houston-Miller N, Schwartz RG. Early return to work after uncomplicated myocardial infarction: results of a randomised trial. *Journal of the American Medical Association* 1988;**260**:214–20.

15. Bertie J, King A, Reed N, Marshall AJ, Ricketts C. Benefits and weaknesses of a cardiac rehabilitation programme. *Journal of the Royal College of Physicians of London* 1992;**26**:147–51.

16. Perk J, Hedback B, Engvall J. Effects of cardiac rehabilitation after coronary artery bypass grafting on readmissions, return to work, and physical fitness: a case-control study. *Scandinavian Journal of Social Medicine* 1990;**18**:45–51.

17. Danchin N, Goepfert PC. Exercise training, cardiac rehabilitation and return to work in patients with coronary artery disease. *European Heart Journal* 1988;**9**:43–6.

18. O'Connor GT, Burning JE, Yusuf S, Goldhaber SZ, *et al.* An overview of randomised controlled trials of rehabilitation with exercise after myocardial infarction. *Circulation* 1989;**80**:234–44.

19. Olsson G, Levin LA, Rehnqvist N. Economic consequences of post-infarction prophylaxis with beta blockers: cost effectiveness of metoprolol. *British Medical Journal* 1987;**294**:339–42.

20. Cummings SR, Rubin SM, Oster G. The cost effectiveness of counseling smokers to quit. *Journal of the American Medical Association* 1988;**261**:75–9.

21. Hugenholz PG. On jumbo and 'junkie' trials. A fumbled affair, a jungle or the ultimate solution? *International Journal of Cardiology* 1991;**33**:1–4.

22. Goldman L, Sai STB, Cook EF, Rutherford JD, Weinstein MC. Cost-effectiveness of routine long-term beta adrenergic antagonist therapy following acute myocardial infarction. *New England Journal of Medicine* 1988;**319**:152–7.

23. Edelson JT, Weinstein MC, Tosteson ANA, Williams L, *et al.* Long-term cost-effectiveness of various initial monotherapies for mild to moderate hypertension. *Journal of the American Medical Association* 1990;**263**:408–13.

24. Goldman L, Weinstein MC, Goldman PA, Williams LW. Cost-effectiveness of HMG-CoA reductase inhibition for primary and secondary prevention of coronary heart disease. *Journal of the American Medical Association* 1991;**265**:1145–51.

25. Kinosian BP, Eisenberg JM. Cutting into cholesterol. Cost-effective alternatives for treating hypercholesterolemia. *Journal of the American Medical Association* 1988;**259**:2249–54.

26. Goel V, Deber RB, Detsky AS. Non ionic contrast media: economic analysis and health policy development. *Canadian Medical Association Journal* 1989;**140**:389–95.

8 Guidelines and audit standards

Report of a workshop held jointly by the Royal College of Nursing Institute, the British Cardiac Society, and the Research Unit of the Royal College of Physicians of London
Prepared on behalf of the joint workshop by:

David Thompson
Professor of Nursing, School of Health, University of Hull

Gerald Bowman
Research Fellow, School of Health, University of Hull

Alison Kitson
Director, Royal College of Nursing Institute, Oxford

David de Bono
Professor of Cardiology, School of Medicine, University of Leicester

Anthony Hopkins
Director, Research Unit, Royal College of Physicians of London

Cardiac rehabilitation has been defined by the World Health Organisation as:

> the sum of activities required to influence favourably the underlying cause of the disease, as well as to ensure the patients the best possible physical, mental and social conditions so that they may, by their own efforts, preserve or resume when lost, as normal a place as possible in the life of the community.[1]

An older, but essentially similar, definition is:

> a process by which a patient is returned realistically to his greatest physical, mental, social, vocational and economic usefulness and, if employable, to employment in a competitive industrial world.[2]

The *necessity* for rehabilitation, as so defined, is unarguable; the *process* by which rehabilitation is achieved has been the subject of much argument and controversy, particularly with regard to the benefit or otherwise of specific rehabilitation programmes. Many of the crucial issues in cardiac rehabilitation have previously been identified in the report of a British Cardiac Society working party.[3]

This chapter summarises the findings of a multidisciplinary

workshop convened to prepare clinical guidelines and audit standards in cardiac rehabilitation held under the joint auspices of the Royal College of Nursing Institute, the Joint Medical Practice and Audit Committee of the British Cardiac Society, and the Royal College of Physicians of London. The workshop developed a three-element model of the rehabilitation process, identified needs relating to medical and psychosocial care, and the potential contributions of education, exercise, secondary prevention and vocational advice. Draft audit standards are proposed as a basis for locally developed guidelines and further research.

In accordance with a convention established in previous workshops, issues which are potential audit points are identified by (A), consensus agreement points by (C), and potential topics for future research by (R). Where there is clear evidence of effectiveness, a statement is followed by a conventional reference.

The rehabilitation process

The time course of cardiac rehabilitation can be divided into four phases:

- *Phase I:* in-hospital,

- *Phase II:* early post-discharge,

- *Phase III:* later post-discharge, and

- *Phase IV:* long-term follow-up.

These phases are spanned by three essential elements, which are interlinked and may be overlapping:

- *Element 1:* the process of explanation and understanding. This should start simultaneously with the process of medical diagnosis and management. Its aim is to ensure that patients at all times have an accurate and up-to-date understanding of what has happened to them, with the implications conveyed sympathetically and positively in readily understandable terms. This has traditionally been regarded as an integral part of good medical and nursing practice, but nevertheless falls within the definition of rehabilitation, and is of such importance that it needs to be audited (A).

- *Element 2:* specific rehabilitation interventions including, where appropriate, secondary prevention, exercise training and psychological support — all tailored to the needs of the individual patient and the setting of the specific medical diagnosis. These interventions are usually applied for a defined period corresponding to the immediate and later phases of post-hospital rehabilitation. The desired outcomes are capable of being specified and measured.

■ *Element 3:* the long-term process of re-adaptation and re-education, and maps to the long-term or open-ended final period of rehabilitation.

The scope of cardiac rehabilitation

Rehabilitation is an intrinsic part of the management of all cardiac disease. Most formal rehabilitation programmes have concentrated on patients recovering from myocardial infarction (MI) or who have had open-heart surgery, based on the perception that these are groups with the maximum potential for health gain. The selection criteria for some programmes for this type of patient mean in fact that patients already in an excellent prognostic category are chosen for rehabilitation, and the 'added value' in these patients will be small. Conversely, patients with heart failure, valvular heart disease, angina and hypertension may also have a large potential for health gain, and could be helped by targeted rehabilitation programmes (R). Such programmes may need to take account of the special needs of the elderly, different ethnic groups, and both genders (R). All too often, the uptake of rehabilitation is lowest among those who could benefit most.

The components of cardiac rehabilitation

Medical diagnosis and intervention

Risk stratification is important, both to define high-risk subgroups and as a basis for more intensive diagnostic efforts. High-risk subgroups may require specific resources and precautions, but sometimes offer an opportunity for high 'health gain'. The role of exercise testing, radionuclide studies and other investigations in risk stratification of patients with angina or following infarction has been discussed in detail elsewhere.[3-5] Exercise testing after MI has a high predictive accuracy[6,7] (ie patients with a negative exercise test at a good workload have an excellent prognosis), and this information can be of great psychological benefit (C). The specific role of exercise testing as a guide to exercise in rehabilitation will be discussed later.

Detailed discussion of interventions, whether surgical (valve replacement, coronary bypass graft, angioplasty) or pharmacological (aspirin, beta-adrenoceptor antagonists, angiotensin-converting enzyme inhibitors, cholesterol lowering agents) is outside the scope of this chapter. Despite good evidence of effectiveness of secondary prevention measures in high-risk cases,[8-10] implementation of pharmacological secondary prevention is still very weak (R,A). Possible reasons and solutions will be discussed later.

Psychosocial care

Psychological consequences may stem from an attempt to adapt to changes brought about by cardiac disease, and are not necessarily related either to infarct size or to any other measurable cardiac status.[11,12] The main psychological goals are to improve quality of life and to aid secondary prevention. These goals can be achieved through the identification and treatment of psychological distress and psychiatric illness, by restoring confidence, and by helping patients to initiate and maintain lifestyle changes.

In most patients, psychological reactions are transient, but there is persistent depression and anxiety in about one-quarter of patients and their partners. These symptoms are easily measured, and usually respond well to simple counselling aimed at addressing their main concerns and correcting misconceptions.[13] Conversely, early careful and consistent explanation can reduce the development of these complications. The main purpose of counselling should be to encourage behavioural change rather than simply to provide emotional support.

Specific steps to improve psychological care in the context of hospital inpatients include:

- psychological assessment within three days of admission using a simple nurse-administered assessment tool (A),[14]

- a clear written statement of health improvement goals at the time of hospital discharge (A).

Cardiac disease disrupts families, and particularly affects partners and carers. Social factors can impinge on recovery: for example patients' and partners' beliefs about the causation of an illness will determine their emotional and practical responses.[15] Patients should be encouraged to remain independent and to have a say in what they are willing to do (autonomy). Relationships in the home, finances, and changes in work and social activity may create problems which are difficult to resolve. Strong partner support is possibly the single most important factor in buffering these effects.[16] After discharge from hospital, less general information about disease and more specific advice about activity is appropriate.[17] The family should be offered participation in all aspects of rehabilitation. Group discussions with patients and partners offer opportunities for comparisons and shared experience, and may be more cost-effective.

Exercise

Supervised physical exercise has traditionally been a central component of cardiac rehabilitation, for several reasons:

1. It is believed that supervised exercise will help restore more rapidly the patient's confidence, feeling of well-being and level of physical activity.

2. It is hoped that increased physical activity will help reverse adverse risk factors and contribute to secondary prevention.

3. Exercise may act as a core activity which provides a vehicle for psychological and social support and for other secondary prevention activities.

Most patients experience a spontaneous improvement in functional capacity over the first few months after an MI which does not seem related to previous activity levels.[18,19] Patients who exercise achieve their optimum functional state more rapidly than patients who do not,[20,21] have fewer visits to their doctors and hospitals,[22] and are more likely to return to work.[23] Patients with angina can benefit from exercise training by experiencing fewer symptoms and increased exercise capacity,[24,25] and patients with impaired left ventricular function have reported symptomatic improvement after exercise training.[26] Some patients with congestive heart failure may show improved functional capacity after exercise training, but results are unpredictable in individual patients.[27,28] The main contraindications to exercise are susceptibility to exercise-induced arrhythmias and unstable angina.

There is extensive epidemiological evidence that increased physical exercise is associated with a lower risk of atherosclerotic heart disease,[29,30] but individual intervention studies have either lacked power to demonstrate a 'hard end-point' benefit or been confounded by other interventions besides exercise. A recent meta-analysis of trials suggests a potential overall mortality reduction of about 20%.[31] The potential interaction between exercise and other secondary prevention measures, including better control of diabetes and the correction of adverse lipid and prothrombotic profiles, needs further research (R).

Types of exercise which improve cardiovascular fitness are now well characterised:

- moderate rather than high-intensity exercise (eg brisk walking) sustained for periods of about 20 min and repeated regularly (C);[32]

- high-intensity exercise may have a role in a minority of patients (eg those returning to strenuous jobs), but requires careful supervision.

If increased exercise levels are to carry over from specific rehabilitation programmes into longer-term unsupervised daily living, the resource implications need to be considered of heavily facility-dependent activities or those which require much travelling or special clothing. Low-risk patients may move rapidly to unsupervised exercise with regular (eg telephone) support and education about a healthy exercise pattern.

Pre-exercise assessment is important both in devising appropriate exercise programmes and for detecting potential risks. Formal treadmill exercise testing is useful for this and also to monitor progress. Elderly patients or those with arthritis, heart failure or respiratory disease may find treadmill testing difficult, and bicycle ergometry may be useful. Other possible simple alternatives include timed corridor or shuttle walk tests. Before discharge from hospital, patients can be taught simple ways of self-assessing the level of physical activity achieved, such as pulse rate measurement and the Borg perceived exertion scale.[33] Exercise prescription needs to be individualised to take into account both the underlying disease and the patient's own requirements and targets. Inability to keep up with an exercise programme may indicate a need for medical reassessment.

Education

In-hospital education programmes for patients and partners improve knowledge,[34,35] reduce anxiety and depression, and decrease disability.[36] With increased trends towards outpatient management and early discharge, similar outpatient facilities are needed (R). Staff should have clear, specific items for discussion covering the diagnosis and its implications, medication and its effects, and available support when needed (A). Coordination is required to avoid conflicting advice. Written and taped information should back up verbal communication[37] and, if required, be available in appropriate languages and Braille. Educational impact can be increased by using a variety of formats and media.

Vocational assessment

Return to work is considered a major end-point in cardiac rehabilitation. Although 62–92% of patients who are working prior to MI return to work,[38] a high proportion leave work again or change jobs in the first year after their return. The patient's attitude towards resuming employment in the acute phase of the illness is a powerful predictor of subsequent return to work. Except for patients with persisting angina or heart failure, failure to return to work is more often due to psychological or financial considerations than to statutory or physical constraints. Even in occupations where health standards are prescribed by statute, there is an increasing move towards individual assessment of risk and capacity and away from arbitrary standards.[39,40] There needs to be collaboration between cardiac rehabilitation and occupational health medicine to ensure optimum and effective return to work.

The cost-effectiveness of cardiac rehabilitation

There seem to be no cost-effectiveness studies of the comprehensive cardiac rehabilitation process as defined above (R). A number of studies, principally from the US, have looked at specific outpatient exercise-based programmes, but the designs of most of them are suspect and the results ambiguous. In general, these studies have shown that medical costs are marginally lower, and patient income greater, in patients who participate in rehabilitation programmes,[41–43] and that quality of life is also improved.[43] Chua and Lipkin concluded in a recent review[44] that:

> cardiac rehabilitation programmes are cost-effective and should be made available to all who would benefit.

Several secondary prevention interventions are regarded as cost-effective, but are not applied to the whole of the population who might benefit. Proper cost-effectiveness assessments of integrated rehabilitation programmes are urgently needed.

The setting of cardiac rehabilitation

Cardiac rehabilitation is a multidisciplinary process which crosses traditional boundaries between hospital and general practice, and between hospital specialties. Provision for cardiac rehabilitation under the UK National Health Service is very variable, and there is little consistency about funding, scope of rehabilitation programmes or audit.[3] A perception that 'cardiac rehabilitation is not effective' is often advanced as a reason for lack of investment.

Responsibility for its provision

The workshop agreed that responsibility for rehabilitation is as follows:

- *Phase I:* responsibility rests with everyone who deals with or cares for cardiac patients, whether in a hospital or primary care setting. There is scope for coordination of approach and for clinical audit at practice, unit or district level.

- *Phases II and III* require facilities best provided and coordinated at secondary care level. Every hospital caring for cardiac patients should have a policy for cardiac rehabilitation, and an organisation to implement it, with both open to audit. The rehabilitation team should include a designated clinician to provide medical input and also to liaise with clinical colleagues. Funding should be explicitly agreed with purchasers and linked to agreed performance indicators.

- *Phase IV:* responsibility falls largely within the primary care setting, but there should be continuing support and feedback from secondary care. Ideally, standards and audit points should be agreed on a district-wide basis.

Clinical standards

Essential points relating to clinical standards are listed below. (Audit proformas are included in the appendices.)

Medical care

1. Patients and, where appropriate, partners and carers should receive accurate and understandable information about medical findings and proposed management.

2. Patients should routinely be assessed for risk factors as part of inpatient or outpatient management, and be given clear advice on risk factor correction.

3. Evidence-based secondary prevention measures should be instituted and recorded.

Psychosocial care

1. Patients admitted to hospital with acute cardiac events should have a simple formal assessment for depression/anxiety before discharge. Where this indicates a potential problem, patients should have access to appropriate treatment/counselling and to follow-up assessment. Partners should be invited to counselling sessions.

2. Patients should have access to expertise as needed (eg psychiatrist/clinical psychologist, vocational counsellor, smoking counsellor).

Exercise

1. Patients with a diagnosis of MI, unstable angina or heart failure should have a recorded assessment of exercise capacity before hospital discharge. Where appropriate, this could be based on a clinical or a simple walking assessment rather than on a formal treadmill test.

2. Patients should have access to a personal exercise plan that can be monitored either in a group setting or at home.

3. Patients should be medically assessed before embarking on an exercise-based rehabilitation programme.

Education

Patients should have access to information relevant to their medical condition and health status. Information may be provided verbally, by printed material, education classes or group discussions. Differing patient requirements should be catered for.

Contracting for cardiac rehabilitation

Purchaser/provider contracts for cardiac rehabilitation need to specify:

- the scope of the contract (all cardiac diagnoses or selected diagnoses, whether access will be open or limited to hospital referrals);

- the selection criteria (if any) to be used and who will apply them;

- the type of services to be offered (ideally, a comprehensive service); and

- whether the commitment to individual patients is to be fixed-term or open ended.

The level of clinical involvement also needs to be specified, and contractors will need to be satisfied about arrangements for a 'seamless' transition between hospital and community.

References

1. World Health Organisation. *Needs and action priorities in cardiac rehabilitation and secondary prevention in patients with CHD.* Geneva: WHO Regional Office for Europe, 1993.

2. Benton JG, Rusk HA. The patient with cardiovascular disease and rehabilitation: the third phase of medical care. *Circulation* 1953;**8**:417–26.

3. Horgan J, Bethell H, Carson P, Davidson C, *et al.* Working party report on cardiac rehabilitation. *British Heart Journal* 1992;**67**:412–8.

4. de Bono DP, Hopkins A. Investigation and management of stable angina: clinical guidelines and audit standards. *Journal of the Royal College of Physicians of London* 1993;**27**:267–73.

5. de Bono DP, Hopkins A. The management of acute myocardial infarction: guidelines and audit standards. *Journal of the Royal College of Physicians of London* 1994;**28**:312–8.

6. Murray RG. Which patients should have exercise testing after myocardial infarction treated with thrombolysis? *British Heart Journal* 1993;**70**:399–400.

7. Cross SJ, Lee HS, Kenmure A, Walton S, Jennings K. First myocardial infarction in patients under 60 years old: the role of exercise tests and symptoms in deciding whom to catheterise. *British Heart Journal* 1993;**70**:428–32.

8. Eccles M, Bradshaw C. Use of secondary prophylaxis against MI in the north of England. *British Medical Journal* 1991;**302**:91–2.

9. Whitford DL, Southern AJ. Audit of secondary prophylaxis after myocardial infarction. *British Medical Journal* 1994;**309**:1268–9.

10. Northridge DB, Shandall A, Rees A, Buchalter M. Inadequate management of hyperlipidaemia after coronary bypass surgery shown by medical audit. *British Heart Journal* 1994;**72**:466–7.

11. Kallio V, Cay E. *Rehabilitation after myocardial infarction. The European experience.* Copenhagen: WHO Regional Office for Europe, 1985.

12. Ladwig KH, Lehmacher W, Roth R, Breithardt G, *et al.* Factors which provoke post infarction depression: results from the post-infarction late potential (PILP) study. *Journal of Psychosomatic Research* 1992;**36**:723–9.

13. Thompson DR. *Counselling the coronary patient and partner.* London: Scutari, 1990.

14. Lewin B, Robertson IH, Cay EL, Irving JB, Campbell M. Effects of self-help post-myocardial infarction rehabilitation on psychological adjustment and use of health services. *Lancet* 1992;**339**:1036–40.

15. Maeland JV, Havik OE. After the myocardial infarction. A medical and psychological study with emphasis on perceived illness. *Scandinavian Journal of Rehabilitation Medicine* 1989;**22**(Suppl):1–87.

16. Miller P, Wikoff R, MacMahon M, Garrett M, *et al.* Personal adjustments and regime compliance one year after myocardial infarction. *Heart and Lung* 1989;**18**:339–46.

17. Doherty ES, Power PW. Identifying the needs of coronary patients' wife-caregivers: implications for social workers. *Health and Social Work* 1990;**15**:291–9.

18. Wohl AJ, Lewis HR, Campbell W, Karlsson E, *et al.* Cardiovascular function during early recovery from acute myocardial infarction. *Circulation* 1977;**56**:931–7.

19. DeBusk RF, Houston N, Haskell W, Fry G, Parker M. Exercise training soon after myocardial infarction. *American Journal of Cardiology* 1979;**44**:1223–9.

20. Hung J, Gordon EP, Houston N, Haskell WL, *et al.* Changes in rest and exercise myocardial perfusion and left ventricular function 3 to 26 weeks after clinically uncomplicated acute myocardial infarction: effects of exercise training. *American Journal of Cardiology* 1984;**54**:943–50.

21. Greenland P, Chu JS. Efficacy of cardiac rehabilitation services: with emphasis on patients after myocardial infarction. *Annals of Internal Medicine* 1988;**109**:650–63.

22. Ades PA, Huang D, Weaver SO. Cardiac rehabilitation participation predicts lower rehospitalization costs. *American Heart Journal* 1992;**123**:916–21.

23. Boudrez II, De Backer G, Comhaire B. Return to work after myocardial infarction: results of a longitudinal population based study. *European Heart Journal* 1994;**15**:32–6.

24. Todd IC, Ballantyne D. Effect of exercise training on the total ischaemic burden as assessed by 24 hour ambulatory electrocardiographic monitoring. *British Heart Journal* 1992;**68**:560–6.

25. Ehsani AA, Biello DR, Schultz J, Sobel BE, Holloszy JO. Improvement of left ventricular contractile function by exercise training in patients with coronary artery disease. *Circulation* 1986;**74**:350–8.

26. Sullivan MJ, Higginbotham MB, Cobb FR. Exercise training in patients with severe left ventricular dysfunction: hemodynamic and metabolic effects. *Circulation* 1988;**78**:506–15.

27. Tristani FE, Hughes CV, Archibald DG, Sheldahl LM, *et al.* Safety of graded symptom-limited exercise testing in patients with congestive heart failure. *Circulation* 1987;**76**:V154–8.

28. Hedback B, Perk J. Can high-risk patients after myocardial infarction participate in comprehensive cardiac rehabilitation? *Scandinavian Journal of Rehabilitation Medicine* 1990;**22**:15–20.

29. Paffenbarger RS, Hyde RT. Exercise in prevention of coronary heart disease. *Preventive Medicine* 1984;**13**:3–22.

30. Rodriguez BL, Curb JD, Burchfield CM, Abbott RD, *et al.* Physical activity and 23 year incidence of coronary heart disease morbidity and mortality among middle-aged men. The Honolulu Heart Program. *Circulation* 1994;**89**:2540–4.

31. O'Connor GT, Buring JE, Yusuf S, Goldhaber SZ, *et al.* An overview of randomized trials of rehabilitation with exercise after myocardial infarction. *Circulation* 1989;**80**:234–44.

32. Stensel DJ, Brooke-Wavell K, Hardman AE, Jones PRM, Norgan NG. The influence of a 1-year programme of brisk walking on endurance fitness and body composition in previously sedentary men aged 42–59 years. *European Journal of Applied Physiology* 1994;**68**:531–7.

33. Borg G. Psychophysical bases of perceived exertion. *Medicine and Science in Sports and Exercise* 1982;**14**:377–81.

34. Steele JM, Ruzicki R. An evaluation of the effectiveness of cardiac teaching during hospitalisation. *Heart and Lung* 1987;**16**:301–11.

35. Raleigh EH, Odtohan BC. The effect of a cardiac teaching program on patient rehabilitation. *Heart and Lung* 1987;**16**:311–7.

36. Hogan CA, Neill WA. Effect of a teaching programme on knowledge, physical activity and socialisation in patients disabled by stable angina pectoris. *Journal of Cardiac Rehabilitation* 1983;**2**:379–84.

37. Lindsay C, Jennrich JA, Biernolt M. Programmed instruction booklet for cardiac rehabilitation teaching. *Heart and Lung* 1991;**20**:648–53.

38. Shanfield SB. Return to work after acute myocardial infarction: a review. *Heart and Lung* 1990;**19**:109–16.

39. Irving JB, Petch MB. Fitness to drive: updated guidelines for cardio-vascular fitness in vocational drivers. *Health Trends* 1994;**26**:38–40.

40. Joy M. Cardiology aspects of aviation safety — the new European perspective. *European Heart Journal* 1992;**13**(Suppl H):21–6.

41. Picard MH, Dennis C, Schwartz RG, Ahn DK, *et al.* Cost-benefit analysis of early return to work after uncomplicated myocardial infarction. *American Journal of Cardiology* 1989;**63**:1308–14.

42. Levin LA, Perk J, Hedback B. Cardiac rehabilitation — a cost analysis. *Journal of Internal Medicine* 1991;**230**:427–34.

43. Oldridge N, Furlong W, Feeny D, Torrance G, *et al.* Economic evaluation of cardiac rehabilitation soon after myocardial infarction. *American Journal of Cardiology* 1993;**72**:154–61.

44. Chua TP, Lipkin DP. Cardiac rehabilitation should be available to all who would benefit. *British Medical Journal* 1993;**306**:731–2.

Appendix

Workshop participants

HN Bethell, *General Practitioner, Alton, Hants*

GS Bowman, *Research Fellow, School of Health, University of Hull*

*EL Cay, *Consultant in Rehabilitation Medicine, Astley Ainslie Hospital, Edinburgh*

+DP de Bono, *Professor of Cardiology, School of Medicine, University of Leicester*

P Doyle, *Senior Medical Officer, Department of Health, London*

*M Edwards, *Chairman, Support Group, Central Middlesex Hospital, London*

*A Gray, *Director, Health Economics Research Centre, Institute of Health Sciences at Wolfson College, Oxford*

*AE Hardman, *Reader in Human Exercise Metabolism, Department of Physical Education, Sports Science and Recreation Management, Loughborough University*

+A Hopkins, *Director, Research Unit, Royal College of Physicians of London*

JH Horgan, *Consultant Cardiologist, Beaumont Hospital, Dublin*

*M Joy, *Consultant Cardiologist, St Peter's Hospital, Chertsey*

AL Kitson, *Director, Royal College of Nursing Institute, Oxford*

*R Lewin, *Professor of Rehabilitation, School of Health, University of Hull*

*A McLeod, *Consultant Cardiologist, Poole Hospital, Poole*

P Milston, *Senior Lecturer in Occupational Therapy, St Martin's College, Lancaster*

*A Radley, *Reader in Health and Social Relations, Department of Social Sciences, Loughborough University*

H Stokes, *Research and Development Fellow, Royal College of Nursing Institute, Oxford*

DR Thompson, *Professor of Nursing, School of Health, University of Hull*

M Thorogood, *Senior Lecturer in Health Promotion Sciences, London School of Hygiene and Tropical Medicine*

I Todd, *Consultant in Rehabilitation Medicine, Astley Ainslie Hospital, Edinburgh*

S Turner, *Cardiac Rehabilitation Coordinator, Alton, Hants*

*Individuals who prepared background papers
+Chairmen

Appendix
Audit proformas

NOTES CONCERNING THE PATIENT AUDIT SHEET

Cardiac rehabilitation is a comparatively new adjunct to the medical treatment of patients with heart disease. Information concerned with cardiac rehabilitation may not always be readily available in the medical notes as this is a multidisciplinary activity that, in the main, takes place on an outpatient basis. It would, therefore, be prudent to discuss this audit with the cardiac rehabilitation coordinator in order to establish the sources of information. The notes below refer to the numbers on the audit sheets.

1.	These audit points determine the primary reason for inclusion in cardiac rehabilitation. The patient code number should be associated only with this exercise, and should not be traceable. The information needed to complete this section will be available in the medical notes.
2.	These audit points address whether coronary risk factors have been assessed. Blood pressure will be measured in mmHg. High- and low-density lipoproteins or total serum cholesterol may be used to determine blood fats. Smoking may be assessed by the volume of cigarettes/pipe tobacco consumed over a period of time or by expired carbon monoxide. Blood sugar is measured in mmol/l and urine sugar as a percentage. Weight is measured in kilograms, and height in metres and millimetres, from which body mass index can be determined. The patient's usual exercise pattern needs to be ascertained. Most of the factors can be found recorded in the patient's medical notes, but the exercise pattern may be documented elsewhere, for example, in the cardiac rehabilitation notes.
3.	These audit points will indicate who is offered exercise testing. Exercise may be tested simply by walking at a particular pace over time, or by a fixed exercise or treadmill test. This information may be available in the medical notes or kept with the exercise technician or cardiac rehabilitation coordinator.
4.	These audit points determine whether the patient has received instructions concerning health behaviour change. There is no standard means of recording this information; local custom and practice will need to be established. This information may be held in the nursing notes or kept with the cardiac rehabilitation coordinator.
5.	These audit points address the exercise programme. The type of programme offered to the patient should be identified together with the frequency of attendance. There is no standard, agreed method of recording this information. The source of this information is likely to be the person responsible for the exercise component or the cardiac rehabilitation coordinator.
6.	These audit points address psychological adjustment. The objective is to determine whether this has been accounted for in the patient's recovery. This may be presented as a subjective impression in the medical notes, for example, as a reference to 'mood', 'anxiety' or 'depression'. A more objective means of determining this may be obtained by using the Hospital Anxiety and Depression scale. The scores will be kept on a separate chart either in the medical notes or retained by the cardiac rehabilitation coordinator.
7.	These audit points address the educational and behavioural opportunities offered to the patient. The objective is to determine the range of strategies available to educate and support the patient's health goals. An educational package may include a number of elements, such as providing literature, individual instruction, group discussion or formal lectures. Most of these activities will take place on an outpatient basis, and will invariably be organised by the cardiac rehabilitation coordinator from whom this information may be obtained.
8.	These audit points establish whether the patient has had certain major medical interventions during rehabilitation. This information will be readily available in the medical assessment and radiological sections of the patient's medical notes.

Abbreviations used in audit proformas
CABG = coronary bypass graft
CPR = cardiopulmonary resuscitation
MI = myocardial infarction
OPD = outpatient department
PTCA = percutaneous transluminal angioplasty

CARDIAC REHABILITATION

PATIENT

1 Initiating event

Angina ☐   MI ☐   Cardiac surgery ☐   Angioplasty ☐   Heart failure ☐

Patient code number ☐

Non-cardiac (specify) ☐

Initiating event date: Month ☐☐   Year ☐☐   Age ☐☐   Gender ☐

Ethnic group (specify) ☐

2 Risk factor assessment

Do the notes contain a record of blood pressure?   Yes ☐ No ☐
Do the notes contain a record of blood fats?   Yes ☐ No ☐
Do the notes contain a record of smoking habits?   Yes ☐ No ☐
Do the notes contain a record of blood or urine sugar?   Yes ☐ No ☐
Do the notes contain a record of both weight and height?   Yes ☐ No ☐
Do the notes contain a record of habitual exercise pattern?   Yes ☐ No ☐

3 Exercise capacity

Do the notes contain a record of exercise capacity being assessed?   Yes ☐ No ☐
Do the notes contain a record of the patient having an exercise test?   Yes ☐ No ☐

4 Personal plan

Do the notes contain a record of the patient being given a written personal rehabilitation plan?   Yes ☐ No ☐
If yes, do the notes contain a copy of the written personal rehabilitation plan?   Yes ☐ No ☐
Do the notes contain a record of smoking habits?   Yes ☐ No ☐
Do the notes contain a record of whether the patient smokes?   Yes ☐ No ☐
If yes, do the notes contain a record of specific advice being given about stopping?   Yes ☐ No ☐
Do the notes contain a record of whether the patient has sexual problems?   Yes ☐ No ☐
If yes, do the notes contain a record of referral for sexual counselling?   Yes ☐ No ☐
Do the notes contain a record of whether the patient has work problems?   Yes ☐ No ☐
If yes, do the notes contain a record of referral for vocational counselling?   Yes ☐ No ☐

5 Exercise programme

Do the notes contain a record of exercise advice? Yes ☐ No ☐

If yes, which of the following have been recommended?

To continue activities of daily living ☐ Home-based exercise ☐ Community-based exercise ☐ Hospital-based exercise ☐

Do the notes contain a record of attendance at formal (hospital or community-based) exercise sessions? Yes ☐ No ☐

If yes, what is the estimate of the attendance rate? 100% ☐ 75% ☐ 50% ☐ 25% ☐ 0% ☐

6 Psychological state

Do the notes contain a record of psychological state? Yes ☐ No ☐

Do the notes contain a record of a formal assessment of anxiety and depression? Yes ☐ No ☐

Do the notes contain a record of whether the patient is anxious? Yes ☐ No ☐

Do the notes contain a record of whether the patient is depressed? Yes ☐ No ☐

If yes, do the notes contain a record of referral for assessment/treatment? Yes ☐ No ☐

7 Education and support

Do the notes contain a record of whether the patient and partner have been offered education? Yes ☐ No ☐

Do the notes contain a record of whether the patient and partner have been offered counselling? Yes ☐ No ☐

Do the notes contain a record of whether the patient and partner have been offered stress management? Yes ☐ No ☐

Do the notes contain a record of whether the patient and partner have been offered a home visit? Yes ☐ No ☐

Do the notes contain a record of whether the patient and partner have been offered advice on what to do in an emergency? Yes ☐ No ☐

Do the notes contain a record of whether the patient and partner have been offered CPR training? Yes ☐ No ☐

8 Medical investigations and treatment

Do the notes contain a record of whether the patient is receiving aspirin? Yes ☐ No ☐

Do the notes contain a record of whether the patient has heart failure? Yes ☐ No ☐

If yes, do the notes contain a record of treatment for the heart failure? Yes ☐ No ☐

Since referral to the programme, do the notes contain a record of the following investigations and treatments?

Angiography ☐ Perfusion imaging ☐ Radionuclide ventriculography ☐ Echocardiography ☐

CABG ☐ PTCA ☐ Transplant ☐ Pacemaker ☐

CARDIAC REHABILITATION   PATIENT SUMMARY

Date of summation: Day ☐☐   Month ☐☐   Year ☐☐   Facility ☐   [   ]

1 Initiating event

Number of patients entering programme with: Angina ☐☐   MI ☐☐   Cardiac surgery ☐☐   Angioplasty ☐☐   Heart failure ☐☐   Other ☐☐

Total number ☐☐   Total number of ☐☐   Total number of patients ☐☐   Lowest age ☐☐   Highest age ☐☐
of patients   elderly patients   from ethnic groups
                     of women

Does the proportion of elderly patients reflect the numbers enrolled for cardiac rehabilitation?   Yes ☐   No ☐

Does the proportion of women reflect the numbers enrolled for cardiac rehabilitation?   Yes ☐   No ☐

Does the proportion of patients from ethnic groups reflect the numbers enrolled for cardiac rehabilitation?   Yes ☐   No ☐

2 Risk factor assessment

Number of patients with recorded blood pressure ☐☐☐

Number of patients with recorded blood fats ☐☐☐

Number of patients with recorded smoking ☐☐☐

Number of patients with recorded blood or urine sugar ☐☐☐

Number of patients with recorded weight and height ☐☐☐

Number of patients with recorded habitual exercise pattern ☐☐☐

3 Exercise capacity

Number of patients with recorded assessment of exercise capacity ☐☐☐

Number of patients with recorded exercise test ☐☐☐

4 Personal plan

Number of patients with recorded written personal rehabilitation plan ☐☐☐

Number of patients with copy in notes of written personal rehabilitation plan ☐☐☐

Number of patients with recorded smoking habit ☐☐☐

Number of patients who smoke ☐☐☐

Number of patients with recorded advice to stop smoking ☐☐☐

Number of patients with recorded sexual problems ☐☐☐

Number of patients with recorded sexual problems who have been referred for sexual counselling ☐☐☐

Number of patients with recorded work problems ☐☐☐

Number of patients with recorded work problems who have been referred for vocational counselling ☐☐☐

5 Exercise programme

Number of patients with recorded advice on exercise

Number of patients with recorded advice to continue activities of daily living

Number of patients with recorded advice for home-based exercise

Number of patients with recorded referral to community-based exercise

Number of patients with recorded referral to hospital-based exercise

Number of patients with recorded attendance at formal (hospital or community-based) exercise sessions

Estimated percentage of attendance

100% ☐ 75% ☐ 50% ☐ 25% ☐ 0% ☐

6 Psychological state

Number of patients with recorded psychological state

Number of patients with recorded formal assessment of anxiety and depression

Number of patients with recorded anxiety

Number of patients with recorded depression

Number of patients with recorded referral for assessment/treatment

7 Education and support

Number of patients and partners with a recorded offer of education

Number of patients and partners with a recorded offer of counselling

Number of patients and partners with a recorded offer of stress management

Number of patients and partners with a recorded offer of a home visit

Number of patients and partners with a recorded offer of advice on what to do in an emergency

Number of patients and partners with a recorded offer of CPR training

8 Medical investigations and treatment

Number of patients recorded as receiving aspirin

Number of patients recorded with treatment for heart failure

Number of patients recorded with treatment for heart failure

Number of patients recorded with angiography since referral to programme

Number of patients recorded with perfusion imaging since referral to programme

Number of patients recorded with radionuclide ventriculography since referral to programme

Number of patients recorded with echocardiography since referral to programme

Number of patients recorded with CABG since referral to programme

Number of patients recorded with PTCA since referral to programme

Number of patients recorded with transplant since referral to programme

Number of patients recorded with insertion of pacemaker since referral to programme

CARDIAC REHABILITATION

FACILITY

Date: Day ☐☐   Month ☐☐   Year ☐☐   Facility (specify) ☐

1 General information

	YES	NO
Does the facility have a cardiac rehabilitation programme?	☐	☐
Does the facility have a policy for entry into the cardiac rehabilitation programme?	☐	☐
If yes, are all staff involved in the programme given a copy of the policy?	☐	☐
Is there written information in the OPD concerning referral to cardiac rehabilitation?	☐	☐
Is there written information in other departments concerning referral to cardiac rehabilitation?	☐	☐
Is there a named consultant associated with the cardiac rehabilitation programme?	☐	☐

2 Policy

	YES	NO
Are the following included in the policy?	☐	☐
Specified minimum individual contacts between patient and rehabilitation staff in the first year	☐	☐
Specified frequency of telephone contact	☐	☐
Guidelines on education	☐	☐
Guidelines on exercise	☐	☐
Guidelines on psychological assessment	☐	☐
Guidelines on counselling	☐	☐
Guidelines on exclusion criteria	☐	☐
Guidelines on follow-up	☐	☐

3 Special group attendance

	YES	NO
Is the attendance of elderly patients recorded?	☐	☐
Is the attendance of women recorded?	☐	☐
Is the attendance of patients from ethnic groups recorded?	☐	☐

4 Programme resources

	YES	NO
Is there accommodation for education?	☐	☐
Is there accommodation for counselling?	☐	☐
Is there accommodation in the hospital for supervised exercise sessions?	☐	☐
Is there accommodation in the community for supervised exercise sessions?	☐	☐
Are there resources for all at-risk patients to be exercise tested within 3 months of the initiating event?	☐	☐
Are there resources for patients to continue exercise once formal programmes are completed?	☐	☐
Is there a patient support group?	☐	☐

5 Training protocol

	YES	NO
Is there a training protocol for rehabilitation staff?	☐	☐
If yes, does this include: education?	☐	☐
counselling?	☐	☐
stress management?	☐	☐
advice on what to do in an emergency?	☐	☐
advanced cardiac life support?	☐	☐